Intermittent Fasting for Women – 2 Books in 1

The Only Weight Loss Guide for Women by a Woman. Discover how to Burn Fat, Slow Aging, Balance Hormones and Feel More Attractive!

Weight Loss for Women

The Ultimate Guide for Women to Lose Weight, Burn Fat, Reset their Metabolism, Stop Aging and Live Longer!

By

Nancy Johnson

work can be in any fashion deemed liable for any hardship or damages that may befall them after undertaking information described herein.

Additionally, the information in the following pages is intended only for informational purposes and should thus be thought of as universal. As befitting its nature, it is presented without assurance regarding its prolonged validity or interim quality. Trademarks that are mentioned are done without written consent and can in no way be considered an endorsement from the trademark holder.

Table of Contents

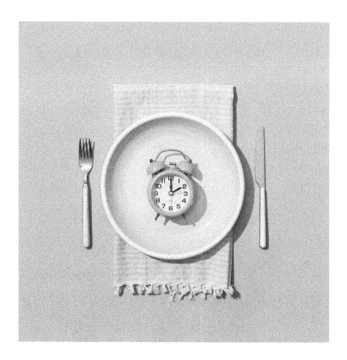

Introduction

Most women over 50 feel as if they have lost their ability to be attractive, healthy and feel good in their own bodies. But what is the cause for this widespread issue? The fact is that in today's world we are spending more and more time at home and we have significantly reduced our need for food. However, even if we do not need as many calories as we did in the past to survive and be healthy, most of us are still eating as if they were running a marathon a day.

Therefore, it should not come as a surprise that most women over 50 years of age are out of shape, overweight and unhealthy. This normally translates into a worse quality of life and is something that is frustrating for a substantial portion of the female population. Thanks to researches and scientific studies conducted by incredible nutritionists, it is now possible to overcome the negative effect of a sedentary life. In fact, intermittent fasting seems like the perfect solution for all those women that want to burn fat, lose weight and gain a healthy and new lifestyle.

The need of all these women is what inspired the writing of this guide. In fact, in the next chapters you are not going to find complicated explanations of scientific topics that, even if interesting, do not give you a clear direction on what you can do to start feeling better. On the contrary, while writing this book, a great effort was made to make sure that each concept is followed by a subsequent strategy that can be implemented in a healthy intermittent fasting protocol.

By reading this book you will get all the information and practical steps you need to follow to start intermittent fasting in just a few days. We advise you to talk to your doctor before changing your diet as intermittent fasting is not suitable if you have certain healthy conditions.

Please, be aware that the goal of this book is to give you accurate information on intermittent fasting, but it does not take the place of a true medical advice. We hope that you can find motivational and informative insights that help you make a change for the better.

Chapter 1 - The most Important Component: Mindset

One of the most important tools at your disposal when you decide to lose weight and win a healthier lifestyle is your ability to make long lasting changes to your routine. In order to do this, you need to have a positive and effective mindset that can sustain you when things get difficult. That is why we have decided to dedicate the first few chapters of this book to this extremely important topic.

The willpower, also known as self-discipline, self-control or determination, is the ability to control your behaviors, emotions and focus. The willpower involves the ability to resist impulses and sacrifice immediate gratification in order to achieve your goals. It also includes the ability to ignore unwelcome thoughts, feelings or impulses, as well as that of self-regulation. The level of willingness of a woman can determine its ability to save for its financial stability, to make positive choices for its mental and physical health and to avoid the use or abuse of harmful substances. Continuing to give up instant gratifications in favor of future prizes, you can move towards your goals and develop your willpower. Thanks to a constant "workout" of the mind, this practice will strengthen your ability to control your impulses, exactly how physical exercise strengthens your muscles.

Let's take a look at some tips that can help you build up your mindset.

Evaluate your habits

If you are trying to improve your willpower, probably your inability to control your impulses is negatively affecting some areas of your life. Some women over 50 struggle with their willpower in every aspect of their life, while others are limited to having some specific "weaknesses". Determine what the area you intend to improve and, if the areas are a lot, choose to dedicate yourself to one at a time.

For example, your willpower could be weak in front of the food. This could consequently negatively affect your health and quality of your life For example, you may have difficulty following your intermittent fasting protocol, which causes you to binge and not be healthy. Whatever health issue you are facing today, acknowledging it is the first step to overcome it.

Create a scale to evaluate your willpower

You will need to evaluate your willpower as efficiently as possible during your intermittent fasting protocol. You could create a scale from 1 to 10, in which 1 represents a complete indulgence relative to the thing, or to things, that you are trying to avoid, and 10 a stoic respect for the restrictive rules that you have established for yourself. Alternatively you can develop a simpler scale, based on "at all, little, more, much". This scale can take different forms, while continuing to offer you the opportunity to evaluate yourself while following an intermittent fasting protocol.

For example, if you realize you eat sweets in a compulsive way or stop in some fast food restaurants on a daily basis, on a scale from 1 to 10 you can evaluate yourself with a 1 or a 2.

Think long term

If you want to improve yourself, the first step to take is to set a goal for your change. You will need to choose a clear, specific and achievable goal. If it were too vague or not measurable, it would indeed be difficult to determine any progress made or establish it achieved.

For example, the "eating healthier" goal, established by those women who tend to eat impulsively, will certainly be too vague. "Healthier" is a relative concept, which will make it difficult to establish when it was reached. A more concrete destination could be to "lose 20 pounds through a healthy intermittent fasting protocol", "return to a size 44" or "overcoming my sugar addiction ".

Have short term goals as well

When you want to reach an important goal (which could appear complicated), one of the best ways to do this is to establish intermediate goals along the way. Your short-term goals must also be specific and measurable, and able to lead you to your final goal.

For example, if you are trying to lose 20 pounds, you can give you a first short-term goal similar to "losing 5 pounds", "do exercise 3 times a week" or "limit desserts to once a week".

Think big

The best way to "train" your willpower is to show you are willing to sacrifice the desire for immediate gratification in favor of a better long-term reward. The final compensation will be that of "living well" or "feeling attractive"; However, to learn how to exercise your willpower it is advisable to establish a concrete prize.

For example, if your desire is to lose weight, trying to control your compulsive hunger through a healthy intermittent fasting protocol, your final reward could be a new dress that makes you feel amazing.

Give up immediate gratification

This is the essence of the development of willpower. When you feel tempted to give up to an impulse, realize that what you really want to live is that short feeling of immediate gratification. In case your impulsive behavior is contrary to your goals, after giving away to immediate gratification you will feel guilty.

To resist the desire for immediate gratification, follow these steps.

- Recognize what you want to do.
- Admit that the only thing you want is immediate gratification.
- Remember your short and long-term goals you set for yourself.
- Ask yourself if it's worth giving to the current impetus and jeopardize your journey towards the ultimate goal.

For example, if you are working to keep nervous hunger under control by following a healthy intermittent fasting protocol and during a party you find yourself in front of a tray full of biscuits, do the following things.

- Feel how much you would like to eat those biscuits.
- Recognize that that biscuit could be able to satisfy your current desire for sweets.
- Remember yourself that you are working to achieve the goal of losing 20 pounds by following intermittent fasting protocol and the reward of a new wardrobe.
- Ask yourself if temporary satisfaction given by that biscuit deserves to renounce the progress made and the potential loss of the final award.

Give yourself small rewards for the results achieved

A motivation or reward system will not change your long-term will strength, but you can help you follow the way to success. Since the achievement of a final goal may take a long time, it could be effective to set small rewards for the progress made so that they act as motivation to keep going.

For example, if for a week you have followed your intermittent fasting protocol, you can give yourself a small dose of your favorite dessert over the weekend. Alternatively, you can reward you with something that is not bound to food, like a pedicure or a massage.

Notes your attempts to check your impulses, including both the successful ones and the unsuccessful ones. Don't forget those details that in the future could help you evaluate the situation.

For example, you could write: "Today I ate five cookies during an office party. I had missed lunch and I was quite hungry. I was surrounded by many people and Sara, who had prepared the cookies, repeatedly encouraged me to eat one of them".

Comment on the factors that influenced your decision-making process

In addition to detailing the situation you have resisted or how you have surrendered to the impulse, describe what has passed through your mind in those moments. You may want to include your emotional state, the people you were next to you and the place where you were there.

After describing several episodes in your diary, you can start to re-read them, trying to highlight possible schemes in your behaviors. Here are some questions you should ask yourself.

- Is my decision-making process more effective when I am alone or when I am with other people?
- Are there some people who more than others "trigger" my compulsive behaviors?
- Do my emotions (depression, anger, happiness, etc.) influence my compulsive behavior?
- Is there a particular moment of the day when it is more difficult to keep my impulses under control?

You can decide to create a visual representation of your progress

It may seem to be a strange idea, but there are many women who respond better to a more concrete visual representation of their progress. It will be easier to remain motivated by having something that clearly shows you the many steps taken so far, as well as those still to be done.

For example, if you want to lose 20 pounds, you can insert a coin in a jar whenever you lose 0,5 lbs. Seeing the level of coins grow while losing weight you will have a concrete representation of the progress made.

Find out what is more effective for you

By reading your diary or simply reflecting on your successes and your false steps, you can realize what is more useful for you. You may notice that giving you a weekly reward is really effective. You could then find that being alone is a triggering cause of your compulsive behavior, or that you find yourself in a given place or in the presence of certain people contribute to increasing your food cravings. Customize your approach to increase your willpower based on your specific needs.

Stress can hinder your progress

Whatever health your goal you are trying to reach, stress deriving from working or personal life has the potential to derail your progress. Therefore, it could be necessary to use techniques to reduce your stress. Do not underestimate the influence stress can have in your ability to follow your intermittent fasting protocol.

Sometimes the best way to defeat temptation is to avoid it. If you feel you don't have the willpower needed to resist your compulsive behavior, try to eliminate the opportunity to give up your intermittent fasting protocol. This could mean wanting to avoid those people or those environments that tend to trigger your cravings. This solution may not be valid long-term, but prove to be useful in the beginning of your intermittent fasting protocol or during some particularly difficult moments.

For example, if you tend to eat outside your scheduled eating window, you can decide to empty your home of all sorts of unhealthy food. Remove from your pantry everything that does not suit your new healthy habits, throwing it away.

Use "if-then" affirmations

You can "mentally feel" your reactions at a given situation by inventing some scenarios in advance using the "if-then" structure. Doing this will be particularly useful when you will find yourself in a situation that tempts you.

For example, if you are about to attend a party where biscuits will be available, you can use the following "if - then" statement. "If Sara will offer me a biscuit, then I gently tell her 'no, thanks, but they look delicious' and I'll move to the other side of the room".

Search for medical help

If you have been trying without success to keep your impulses at bay, evaluate the hypothesis to turn to a therapist. They can offer you support and specific tips to change your behaviors.

People suffering from obsessive or compulsive behavior or dependencies can benefit from the help of a therapist specialized in impulse control disorders or cognitive pathologies.Some impulse control disorders and some deficiencies in the willpower can also benefit from a treatment known as "Habit Reversal Therapy" which replaces unwanted habit with another more useful habit.

Chapter 2 - How to Set Your Goals

Whether you have small dreams or high expectations from your intermittent fasting protocol, having goals will allow you to plan your path through this weight loss journey. The achievement of some goals can require a whole life, while others can be conquered from morning to evening. Whatever your goals, broad and generic or specific and practical, in reaching them you will feel satisfied and you will see your self-esteem grow. If the fulfillment of the first necessary steps intimidates you, continue reading and find out how to consolidate the widest desire.

Determine the goals for your life

Ask yourself important questions regarding what you want to get from life. On a physical level, you might want to be back in shape by following an intermittent fasting protocol.

Analyze the areas in which, over time, you would like to make changes or improvements. Start wondering what you want to get in every specific area, and think about what steps you want to take in the next five years.

In the case of the goal "I want to get back in shape", you could establish minor goals as "I want to follow my intermittent fasting protocol" and "I want to fast at least 16 hours a day".

Once you know what you want to get over the next few years, you have to start taking the steps necessary to reach them by writing down the actual goals.

If you want to get back in shape, your first goal may be to eat more fruits and vegetables and run for 3 miles. We will have a chapter dedicated to writing down your goals in the best possible way, for now just know that it is fundamental if you want to lose weight and keep it off.

You have to highlight the reasons why you have decided to set such a goal and reflect on what will happen once you reach it. For example, if referring to a short-term fitness goal you have decided to achieve, it is good to ask yourself if and how your choice will help you reach your main health goal. If necessary, evaluate to change your short-term goal by replacing it with a practice that allows you to effectively advance towards the final destination.

Periodically check your goals

Instead of limiting you to remain anchored on your initial positions, from time to time find time to re-evaluate your minor goals. Are you respecting the temporal deadlines you have set for yourself? Are the steps planned able to lead you to your finish line? Be flexible in changing and adapting your minor goals.

To get back in shape, you may have to follow an intermittent fasting protocol for several weeks. If you start by following a 16/8 intermittent fasting protocol it might be the case for you to take things to a new level by committing yourself to an 18/6 protocol. Have fixed goals but do not be afraid to change your approach to reach them faster.

Make your goals specific

When you set a goal, you have to make sure that you respond to very specific questions: who, what, where and why. For any goal you set, you should reflect on your reasons and ask you how it helps to get you to achieve what you want in life.

To get back in shape (very generic destination), you should create a more specific goal like following an intermittent fasting protocol for a full month. For every goal you set for yourself, you should be as specific and precise as possible. For instance, an example of a well-built goal could be "I am going to lose 10 lbs in one month by following an intermittent fasting protocol".

Measurable goals

In order to be able to track the progress made, your goals should be measurable. "I'm going to follow an intermittent fasting protocol" is a difficult goal to measure and to track compared to "every day I have only an 8 hour window to eat". In practice, you must be able to determine if you have reached your goal or not.

Be realistic when setting up your goals

It is important to evaluate your situation honestly and distinguish realistic goals from unlikely ones. Ask yourself if you have all the tools needed to reach the set goal.

If you don't have the time or interest needed to dedicate many hours to an intermittent fasting protocol every week, this goal is not for you. If this were your case, it will therefore be necessary to choose an alternative path - there are many ways, in fact, to be able to keep yourself in shape without having to follow an intermittent fasting protocol.

At every moment you will have many goals and at different completion stages. You have to decide which are the most important or urgent ones for you. Being committed to achieving too many goals simultaneously will make you feel overwhelmed and will reduce your chances of success. It can be useful to set some main priorities. In this way, when two goals will come into conflict, you will know how to behave. If the choice will fall between completing one or two minority goals or a priority one, you will have no doubt on what to do.

Keep track of the progress made

Writing in a diary allows you to track your progress, both personal and professional and, when you are directed towards a goal, performing an analysis of the steps taken is a great way to keep you motivated. Analyzing your achievements will be a good source of motivation to do better.

Give the right value to the achievement of your goals

Whenever you reach a goal, you should recognize and celebrate your success as it deserves. Reflect on the path that led you to the goal, from the beginning to the end. Evaluate if the goal has satisfied you, evaluate your new skills and knowledge and note if the goal has been reached in full. Once you have reached your goal, just set another one for yourself to keep building on the momentum you have created.

Now that we have seen how to set good goals for a healthier version of you, it is time to analyze how to actually write them down to make sure you have the highest chance of reaching them. After that, we will finally be able to start talking about the most effective intermittent fasting protocols you can follow to lose weight fast.

Weight Loss for Beginners

Chapter 3 - How to Write Down Your Goals for Maximum Results

As we have seen in the previous chapters, a goal is a mental representation of a specific and measurable result that you want to reach through commitment to certain actions. At its base there may be a dream or hope, but unlike dreams a goal is quantifiable. With a well-written goal, you will know what you want to get and how you intend to get it. Writing personal goals can be both incredibly satisfying and widely useful. Some studies have shown that setting goals for your intermittent fasting protocol can help you feel much safer and confident, even when it comes to long-term fasting periods. As the Chinese philosopher Lao Tzu said: "A thousand miles trip starts with a single step". You can start taking the journey that will take you to the desired destination by writing down your personal weight loss goals.

Reflect on what is considered significant

Studies show that when your goals concern something that you consider motivating, you are more likely to reach them. Identify the areas of your life in which you would like to make changes. In this initial phase, it is normal for every area to have rather large borders. Generally, people decide to give themselves goals in terms of self-improvement and physical health. An accurate intermittent fasting protocol can help you move towards these two directions at the same time.

You should start by drafting out your goals on a piece of paper. For example, you may want to make significant changes in areas concerning health and physical well being. Write down this information, specifying what you would like to change.

At this stage you could indicate the goals in vague terms, it is normal. As for health, for example, you could write "improve physical form" or "healthy eating".

Identify your "best self"

Studies suggest that determining which you think is the best possible version of yourself can help you feel more positive and satisfied with your life. No less important, it is a way to understand what are the goals that you really consider significant. Identifying what is the "best yourself as possible" requires two steps. First of all, you have to see yourself in the future, once you reach your goals, and evaluate what are the qualities you need to get to that point.

Imagine a moment in the future when you have become the best possible version of yourself. How will you be? What things will you give more importance to? At this point, it is essential to concentrate on what "yourself" considers important, ignoring the pressures and desires of others.

Imagine the details of this "future you" and think positive. You can think about something that is the "dream of your life", a fundamental stage of your weight loss journey or some other significant result. For example, your best self could be a healthy woman who follows an intermittent fasting protocol with ease. In this case, imagine what you would do. Which intermittent fasting protocol would you follow? How many calories would you eat per day?

Please, put as many details of your best self when writing down your goals. Imagine what qualities your "best self" is using to achieve success. For example, assuming that you are following an intermittent fasting protocol, surely you would know how to meal prep and manage hunger. Those are two skills you just discovered you must develop to improve your health.

Once you have a list of the skills you need to develop, think about which of these qualities you already have. Be honest with yourself, not severe. Then reflect on the qualities you can develop. Imagine ways to be able to develop the habits and skills you need. For example, if you want to follow an intermittent fasting protocol, but you have no knowledge about eating healthy, you can buy a few books about this topic. The beauty of knowledge is that it can be acquired.

Fix priorities for different areas

Once you have filled out a list of areas in which you would like to make changes, you have to put them in order of priority. Trying to improve all aspects of your life at once is likely to end up with you feeling exhausted, running the risk of failing to achieve your goals because they seem impossible.

Divide your goals in three distinct sections:

- General goals
- Second-level goals
- Third-level goals

The first are the most important, because they are the ones who feel more significant to you. Those of the second and third level are relevant, but you do not give them the same value as the general goals. They also tend to be more specific.

An example might be helpful. At the general level you might want to "give priority to your health by following an intermittent fasting protocol". At the second level you may want to "be a good friend, keep the house clean, and be a good parent". At the third level you might want to "Learn to knit or become more efficient at work".

Start narrowing the field

When you have established what the areas you would like to change are and what changes you would like to make, you can start determining the specifications of what you would like to achieve. These specifications will be the basis of your goals. By answering some questions you will be able to identify the who, the what, the when, the where and the results you want to achieve.

Studies carried out suggest that formulating a specific goal not only increases the chances of being able to reach it, but it also helps you feel more happy about the changes it requires.

Determine the who

When you formulate a goal, it is important to determine who is responsible for achieving every sub-goal. Since we are talking about personal goals, it is very likely that the responsible is you. Nevertheless, some goals require the cooperation of others, so it is useful to identify who will be responsible for those parts.

For example, "following an intermittent fasting protocol" is a personal goal that probably only involves you. Otherwise, if your goal is "helping my entire family follow an intermittent fasting protocol", it will also be necessary to contemplate the responsibility of other people.

Determine the what

Asking yourself this question helps you to define the goal, the details and results you want to get. For example, "following an intermittent fasting protocol" is a goal too wide to be manageable. It lacks precision. Reflect on the details of what you want to learn to do. "Follow an intermittent fasting protocol and lose 10lbs in 5 weeks" is more specific.

The more details you can add to the what, the clearer the steps you will have to take to achieve your goal.

Determine the when

One of the key factors of correctly formulating your goals is to divide them in different stages. Knowing when you have to reach every specific step can help you stay on the right track, while giving you the clear feeling of being progressing.

Be realistic in setting the different stages you want to reach. "Losing five pounds by following an intermittent fasting protocol" is not something that can occur from one week to another. Reflect on how long it is really necessary to reach every stage of your plan.

Determine the where

In many cases, it may be useful to identify a certain place where you will reach your goal. For example, if what you are pursuing is following an intermittent fasting protocol three times a week, it is good to decide if you intend to cook at home, buy food on the go or have it delivered at your house. It might seem useless to write down so many details, but trust us when we say that they can make or break your ability to achieve your goals.

Determine the how

This step urges you to imagine how you intend to reach every stage of the process to your goal. This way you will define the structure more precisely and you will have a clear idea of the actions you have to do to complete each phase.

Returning to the example of the intermittent fasting protocol, you will need to choose a meal plan, get the ingredients, have the necessary tools and find the time to prepare your meals in the kitchen.

Determine the why

As mentioned above, the chances of being able to achieve your goal increase proportionately to how significant and motivating it feels. Determining the reason behind your goal helps you understand what is the motivation that drives you to achieve a certain goal.

In our example, you may want to follow an intermittent fasting protocol to feel more attractive and be healthy.

It is important to keep the "why" in mind while you do the actions necessary to achieve your goals. Giving you highly specific goals is useful, but you also need to always have a clear motivation that pushes you when things get difficult.

Write your goals in positive terms

Research shows that you are more likely to reach your goals if you express them in positive terms. In other words, write them considering them something towards which you are moving, not something you want to avoid.

For example, if one of your goals is to follow an intermittent fasting protocol, a motivating way to express it would be "eat only from 6pm to midnight".

On the contrary, "not eat from midnight to 6pm" is not very encouraging or motivating. Words become things, so be careful in what words you decide to use.

Make sure your goals are based on performance

Succeeding certainly requires hard work and a strong motivation, but you must also be sure of setting goals that your commitment allows you to reach. The only thing you can control is your actions, not those of others and not the results.

Focus your goals on the actions you can do yourself, instead of specific results. By conceiving success as a performance process, you will be able to feel that you have remained faithful to the commitment taken even on the occasions when the result is not the one you hoped.

Define your strategy

These are the actions and tactics you intend to use to achieve your goals. Break down the strategy in individual concrete tasks as it makes it even easier to put yourself into practice. Furthermore, it helps you monitor progress. Use the answers you gave the previous questions (what, where, when etc.) to be able to determine what your strategy is.

Determine the time frame

Some goals can be achieved more quickly than others. For example, "following an intermittent fasting protocol for a day" is something you can start doing immediately. For other goals, instead, you will have to sustain a much longer effort.

Divide your plan in individual tasks

Once you have determined what is the destination you need to reach, and in what time period you have to do it, you can divide your strategy into smaller and concrete tasks. In practice you can determine the individual actions you have to do to reach that goal. Give yourself a deadline for each one of them to know if you are respecting your plans.

Divide these smaller steps into even smaller tasks

By now, you will probably have noticed the tendency to break down every plan into smaller ones. There is a good reason to do this: research has proven that specific goals are more likely to be achieved, even when they are complex. The reason is that it can be difficult to act in the best way when you do not know what you need to do.

Lists the specific actions you are already taking towards your goal

It is likely that you are already behaving or acting in the correct direction. For example, if you wish to follow an intermittent fasting protocol, you might already be skipping breakfast.

Try to be the most specific possible when you create this list. You could realize you have already completed the tasks or duties without even noticing it. This is a very useful exercise that can give you the feeling of being progressing towards the goal.

Identify what skills you need to learn and develop

With regard to many goals, it is likely that you have not yet developed all the qualities or habits that are needed to reach them. Reflect on what skills and habits you can already count on that are useful to your goal. The exercise of the "best possible version of yourself" can be useful in this case as well.

Make a plan for today

One of the main causes why women fail to achieve their weight loss goals is that they think they have to start to pursue them tomorrow. Think of something you can do today to start putting a part of your plans into practice, it doesn't matter if it is a very small action. The action you have completed today can be of a preparatory type for those you will have to do in the following days. For example, you may notice that you have to collect information before making a certain meal plan for your intermittent fasting protocol. You could browse the web and learn how to cook those foods in the best way. Even a small achievement like this one will provide you with a good dose of the motivation you need to continue.

Identify the obstacles

No one likes to think about the obstacles that can prevent them from succeeding, but it is essential to identify the difficulties you could meet when developing your plan to reach your weight loss goal. This step is useful to make you find ready in case something goes differently from how you planned it. Identify the potential obstacles and actions you will have to take to overcome them.

Fear is one of the main obstacles women face when starting an intermittent fasting protocol. The fear of not being able to get what you want can prevent you from taking productive steps that would allow you to achieve success. The next section of the chapter will teach you to fight your fears using some specific techniques.

Use visualization

Research has shown that visualization may have significant effects on improving your performance. Often, athletes claim that visualizing is the technique at the base of their successes. There are two types of visualization

- Visualization of the result
- Visualization of the process

If you want to have the highest probability of succeeding, you should combine them both.

Visualizing the result means imagining to reach your goal. As for the exercise of the "best self", the visualized image should be the most specific and detailed possible. Use all your senses to create this mental photograph: imagine who is there with you, what smells you perceive, what you hear, how you're dressed, where you are. At this stage of the process, it could be useful to build a vision board.

Visualizing the process means imagining the steps you need to take to be able to achieve your goal. Think of all the actions you have undertaken. The psychologists define it as "prospective memory". This process can help you believe that the tasks you face are feasible. In some cases you will even have the feeling of having already completed them with good results.

Use the power of positive thinking

Some studies have shown that, instead of concentrating on defects and errors, thinking positively can help you adapt better to situations, to learn more easily and change effortlessly. No matter what your goal is: thinking positive is as effective for maximum level athletes as for women that want to lose weight.

Some studies have even demonstrated that positive and negative thinking affect different areas of the brain. Positive thinking stimulates areas of the brain associated with visual processing, imagination, the ability to have detached views, empathy and motivation.

For example, remind yourself that your goals are positive growth experiences instead of something that forces you to avoid certain foods or abandon your habits.

If you have difficulty reaching your goals, ask the support of friends and family.

Recognize the "false hope syndrome"

This is an expression with which psychologists describe a cycle that is probably not foreign to you, if you have written a list of resolutions for the new year before. This cycle is composed of three parts: 1) fix the goal, 2) be surprised to find out how difficult it is to reach that goal 3) give up on the goal.

The same cycle can intervene when you expect to get immediate results (which often happens with resolutions for the new year). Fixing specific temporal strategies and deadlines will help you fight these unrealistic expectations.

The same can happen when the initial enthusiasm, which is born when establishing your goals, vanishes and the only thing that remains is the work you need to do to reach them. Formulating strategies and dividing them in smaller tasks can help you keep the momentum you need. Whenever you carry out an assignment, even the smallest one, you can (and you will have to) celebrate your success.

Consider false steps as opportunities to learn more about yourself

The studies carried out show that women who know how to learn from their mistakes have a more positive vision regarding the possibility of achieving their goals. Optimism is a vital component of success. When you are confident you are more likely to be able to look forward instead of backwards.

Research has also shown that the number of false steps committed by those who reach success is neither lower nor higher than those who surrender. The only difference is given by how women choose to consider their mistakes.

Stop searching for perfection

Often, the search for perfectionism originates from the fear of being vulnerable. In many cases we have the desire to "be perfect" to avoid having to face a defeat or a "failure", but the truth is that perfectionism cannot protect us from these experiences, which are completely natural for human beings. The only result you would get would be to impose standards that are impossible to reach. Several studies have confirmed that there is a very strong link between perfectionism and unhappiness.

Be grateful for who you are right now

Research has shown that there is a considerable bond between the active practice of gratitude and the ability to reach your goals. Keeping a diary of gratitude is one of the simplest and most effective methods to learn to feel grateful in everyday life.

It is not necessary to write a lot. Even one or two sentences regarding a person or experience for which you feel grateful will raise the desired effect.

The idea of keeping such a diary could seem silly or childish, but the truth is that the more you believe its power, the more you can feel grateful and happy. Leave the skeptical thoughts out of the door.

Savor specific moments, even those apparently less relevant. Do not hurry to transcribe them into the diary. Take all the time to enjoy the experience, thoroughly reflecting on its meaning and reasons that make you feel grateful. The studies conducted on the subject have shown that to write every day is less effective than just doing it a few times a week. The reason could be that we tend to lose sensitivity to positive things over time, so make sure you maximize the effects of this method.

If you follow these goal setting strategies we are sure you are going to have an advantage over those women that just decide to start an intermittent fasting protocol without the right mindset.

Chapter 4 - The Basics of Nutrition

Now that we have talked about the right mindset you need to achieve your weight loss goals, it is time to study the basics of nutrition. In fact, by understanding how foods behave once they enter your body, you will discover the best way to eat while following an intermittent fasting protocol. Remember that our goal is to help you lose weight while staying healthy. You should never sacrifice your long term health to lose weight faster. This has never worked out well and never will.

During the evolution of the species, humans have undergone a variation of the alimentary patterns due to a multiplicity of factors. From its origin mankind is omnivorous, able to consume a wide variety of plant and animal materials. It is even noted that omnivorism goes back in time, uniting sandwiches and little men to this diet, differentiating them from other evolutionary lines. In this sense, already from the origins Homo is assimilated to the omnivorism of chimpanzees and bonobo, and relatively distant from the vegetarianism of orangutans.

During different phases of the paleolithic the various hominin species employed hunting, fishing and harvesting as primary sources of food, alternating to the spontaneous plants the animal proteins, and preceding in the evolutionary history the finding of such proteins through saprophagous behaviors (ethology widely spread in H. habilis). It has been proven that the genus Homo has used fire since the time of the predominance of the species Homo erectus that of the fire made documented use, probably also for preparing and cooking food before consuming it. According to Lewis Binford, the feeding of animal carrions has extended to later genera than habilis, involving the so-called Peking Man.

The use of fire has become documented regularly in the species H. sapiens and H. neanderthalensis. It is hypothesized, on a scientific basis, that an evolutionary engine for H. erectus, the first hominid documented to be able to cook food was formed by obtaining, with cooking, more calories from the diet, decrease the hours dedicated to the feeding overcoming the metabolic limitations that in the other primates have not allowed an encephalization and a neuronal development tied to the size of the brain in proportion to the body size. This, combined with an increasing consumption of animal proteins, documented to be ascribed to the Homo-Australopithecus separation, or H. habilis-H. erectus, would have been a powerful evolutionary impulse.

Nutrition is a multifaceted process that depends on the integrity of the functions, such as the introduction of food into the oral cavity, chewing, swallowing, digestion, intestinal transit, absorption and metabolism of nutrients. Human nutrition corresponds to the conscious consumption of food and drink; it is influenced by biological, relational, psychological, sensory or socio-cultural factors. In some periods of life as a newborn or elderly, as well as for some pathologies, an organism may not be able to feed itself autonomously, but it needs assistance. In this case we speak of «assisted nutrition».

When the organism is fed by ways that bypass the natural mode, an «artificial nutrition» is carried out. The medical sciences (human and veterinary) deal with the modalities of administration by artificial routes in case of pathologies involving the apparatuses interested in the introduction of food.

Now that we have done this quick historical introduction, let's take a look at the basic elements of nutrition. We are talking about carbohydrates, fats and proteins.

Nancy Johnson

Chapter 5 - Carbohydrates

Carbohydrates are the most common source of energy in living organisms, and their digestion requires less water than protein or fat. Proteins and fats are structural components needed for organic tissues and cells, and are also a source of energy for most organisms. Carbohydrates in particular are the largest resource for metabolism. When there is no immediate need for monosaccharides they are often converted into more space-friendly forms, such as polysaccharides. In many animals, including humans, this form of storage is glycogen, located in liver and muscle cells. The plants instead use starch as a reserve. Other polysaccharides such as chitin, which contribute to the formation of the exoskeleton of arthropods, instead play a structural function. Polysaccharides are an important class of biological polymers. Their function in living organisms is usually structural or depository. Starch (a glucose polymer) is used as a polysaccharide of deposition in plants, and is found both in the form of amylose and in the branched form of amylopectin. In animals, the structurally similar glucose polymer is the most densely branched glycogen, sometimes called "animal starch". The properties of glycogen allow it to be metabolized more quickly, which adapts to the active lives of moving animals. The most common forms of glycogen are hepatic glycogen and muscle glycogen. Hepatic glycogen is found in the liver, it is the reserve of sugar and energy in animals and lasts 24 hours. Muscle glycogen is the reserve of sugar used directly by muscle cells without passing through blood circulation. Hepatic glycogen, on the other hand, must be introduced into the bloodstream before it reaches the cells and, in particular, muscle tissue. Glucose is relevant in the production of mucin, a protective biofilm of the liver and intestine. The liver must be in a state of excellent health to operate the synthesis of missing glucose from proteins, as is required in low-carb diets. Cellulose is located in cell walls and other organisms, and is believed to be the most abundant organic molecule on Earth. The chitin structure is similar, it has side chains that contain nitrogen, increasing its strength. It is found in the exoskeletons of arthropods and in the cell walls of some fungi.

Role in nutrition

A completely carbohydrate-free diet can lead to ketosis. However, the brain needs glucose to draw energy from: this glucose can be obtained from the milk of nuts, an amino acid present in proteins and also from the glycerol present in triglycerides. Carbohydrates provide 3.75 kcal per gram, proteins 4 kcal per gram, and fats provide 9 kcal per gram. In the case of proteins, however, this information is misleading as only some of the amino acids can be used to derive energy. Similarly, in humans, only some carbohydrates can provide energy, including many monosaccharides and disaccharides. Other types of carbohydrates can also be digested, but only with the help of intestinal bacteria. Ruminants and termites can even digest cellulose, which is not digestible by other organisms. Complex carbohydrates which cannot be assimilated by man, such as cellulose, hemicellulose and pectin, are an important component of dietary fibre. Carbohydrate-rich foods are bread, pasta, legumes, potatoes, bran, rice and cereals. Most of these foods are rich in starch. The FAO (Food and Agriculture Organization) and the WHO (World Health Organization) recommend to ingest 55-75% of the total energy from carbohydrates, but only 10% from simple sugars. The glycemic index and glycemic load are concepts developed to analyze the behavior of food during digestion. These classify carbohydrate-rich foods based on the speed of their effect on blood glucose level. The insulin index is a similar, more recent classification that classifies food by its effect on blood insulin levels, caused by various macronutrients, especially carbohydrates and certain amino acids present in food. The glycemic index is a measure of how quickly carbohydrates of food are absorbed, while the glycemic load is the measure that determines the impact of a given amount of carbohydrates present in a meal.

When you follow an intermittent fasting protocol, during the fasting hours your body is depleted from its carbohydrates reserves and uses fat to fuel your movements and thoughts. This is what allows you to literally melt fat once you reach the last few hours of your fast. It is a powerful concept inspired by nature and it works incredibly well for women of your age.

Chapter 6 - Proteins

In chemistry, proteins (or protids) are biological macromolecules made up of amino acid chains bound together by a peptide bond (a link between the amino group of one amino acid and the carboxylic group of the other amino acid, created through a condensation reaction with loss of a water molecule). Proteins perform a wide range of functions within living organisms, including catalysis of metabolic reactions, synthesis functions such as DNA replication, response to stimuli, and transport of molecules from one place to another. Proteins differ from each other especially in their sequence of amino acids, which is dictated by the nucleotide sequence preserved in the genes and which usually results in protein folding and a specific three-dimensional structure that determines its activity.

By analogy with other biological macromolecules such as polysaccharides and nucleic acids, proteins form an essential part of living organisms and participate in virtually every process that takes place within cells. Many are part of the category of enzymes, whose function is to catalyze biochemical reactions vital to the metabolism of organisms. Proteins also have structural or mechanical functions, such as actin and myosin in the muscles and proteins that make up the cytoskeleton, which form a structure that allows the cell to be maintained. Others are essential for inter- and intracellular signal transmission, immune response, cell adhesion and cell cycle. Proteins are also necessary elements in animal nutrition, since they cannot synthesize all the amino acids they need and must obtain the essential ones through food. Thanks to the digestion process, the animals break down the proteins ingested in the individual amino acids, which are then used in the metabolism.

Once synthesized in the organism, proteins exist only for a certain period of time and then are degraded and recycled through cellular mechanisms for the protein turnover process. The duration of a protein is measured in terms of half-life and can be very varied. Some may exist for only a few minutes, others up to a few years. However, the average lifespan in mammalian cells is between 1 and 2 days. Abnormal and misfolded proteins can cause instability if they are not degraded more quickly.

Proteins can be purified from other cellular components using a variety of techniques such as ultracentrifugation, precipitation, electrophoresis and chromatography. The advent of genetic engineering has made possible a number of methods to facilitate such purification. Commonly used methods to study protein structure and function include immunohistochemistry, site-specific mutagenesis, X-ray crystallography, nuclear magnetic resonance imaging. The proteins differ mainly for the sequence of the amino acids that compose them, which in turn depends on the nucleotide sequence of the genes that express the synthesis within the cell.

A linear chain of amino acid residues is called "polypeptide" (a chain of several amino acids bound by peptide bonds). A protein generally consists of one or more long polypeptides that may be coordinated with non-peptide groups, called prosthetic groups or cofactors. Short polypeptides, containing less than about 20-30 amino acids, are rarely considered proteins and are commonly called peptides or sometimes oligopeptides. The sequence of amino acids in a protein is defined by the sequence present in a gene, which is encoded in the genetic code. In general, the genetic code specifies 20 standard amino acids. However, in some organisms the code may include selenocysteine (SEC), and in some archaea, pyrrolysine, and finally a 23rd amino acid, N-formylmethionine, a methionine derivative, which initiates protein synthesis of certain bacteria.

Shortly after or even during protein synthesis, protein residues are often chemically modified by post-translational modification, which if present alters physical and chemical properties, bending, stability, activity and ultimately, the function of the protein. Proteins can also work together to achieve a particular function and often associate in stable multiprotein complexes.

Proteins that contain the same type and number of amino acids may differ from the order in which they are located in the structure of the molecule. This aspect is very important because a minimal variation in the sequence of amino acids of a protein (that is in the order in which the various types of amino acids follow each other) can lead to variations in the three-dimensional structure of the macromolecule which can make the protein non-functional. A well-known example is the case of the human hemoglobin beta chain, which in its normal sequence carries a trait formed by the following proteins: valine-histidine-leucine-threonine-proline-glutamic acid-lysine.

Proteins and nutrition

The biological value of a protein identifies its ability to meet the metabolic needs of the body for total amino acids and essential amino acids.

The protein quality varies according to the digestibility of the protein (% digested amount and amount of amino acids absorbed in the gastrointestinal tract) and its composition in essential amino acids.

Foods of animal origin (meat, cold cuts, fish, eggs, milk and dairy products) have high biological quality proteins because they contain all the essential amino acids in adequate quantities and are easy to digest. For this reason they are also called noble proteins or high biological value .

Cereals (bread, pasta, rice, spelt, etc.) and legumes (chickpeas, peas, soya, beans, etc.), being of vegetable origin, contain proteins with reduced biological value and that is of inadequate quality. In fact, on the one hand they are not digestible, on the other they do not contain, or contain in insufficient quantity, some essential amino acids.

To ensure protein completeness, even by consuming foods of vegetable origin, it is essential to combine cereals and legumes by consuming traditional Mediterranean dishes. We are talking about pasta and beans, legume soups with spelt/barley, rice and peas, etc. These foods, consumed together, provide a good quantity and quality of amino acids similar (but not equal) to food of animal origin.

Protein daily requirement

The daily protein requirement of a subject depends on several factors, such as age, sex, body weight, physiological-nutritional status and physical activity.

It should be remembered that the body does not stock protein, so it is important to meet the daily protein requirement ensuring the correct amount of essential amino acids.
Based on the LARN requirements (Reference Nutrient Intake Levels - IV revision 2014) and the quality of the proteins introduced by the American population, it has been calculated, on average, how much protein should be taken by age, sex, and weight. For women over 50 years of age, it is recommended one gram of protein for every pound of body weight. So, if you are 120 lbs, you should get at least 60 grams of proteins per day.

Correct intake of protein

To fully exploit all the potential of proteins, it is necessary to make an optimal use so that they are not "dispersed" because they are used as energy. The energy needed for the human body must come mainly from carbohydrates and fats, so that only a part of the protein is used as energy. Protein foods, in particular of animal origin, must be consumed at main meals, e.g.:

The so-called dissociated diets, which provide only proteins or only carbohydrates, not only do not work, but, without introducing on every meal carbohydrates and fats, proteins are consumed thus establishing a protein-energy malnutrition. Obviously the energy introduced must respect the energy balance. You have to introduce as much as you consume, otherwise the macronutrients in excess (proteins or fats or carbohydrates) are stored in your belly. Another important factor is low-calorie and high-protein diets. The diet of protein alone must be prescribed by the nutritionist doctor who limits its consumption over time and in the quality of nutrients. High-protein diets, or DIY diets can make you quickly lose a few extra pounds, but they also often consume lean-mass proteins (muscles, etc.) and thereby reduce the metabolic capacity of the body so that when you go back to eating normally, you take back that pounds.

Chapter 7 - Fats

Lipids are an important energy reserve for animals and plants, as they are able to release a large amount of calories per unit mass. The caloric value of one gram of lipids is about twice as high as sugar and protein, about 9.46 kcal/g versus 4.15 kcal/g. That's why they are the ideal energy substrate for cells. In a healthy woman of 120lbs, there are about 25lbs of fat. During physical activity lipids are used together with carbohydrates, providing the same amount of energy for medium-low level activities. If physical activity lasts for at least an hour you encounter a depletion of carbohydrate stocks (glycogen) and a corresponding increase in the use of lipids. In addition, food lipids provide essential fatty acids (that is, not synthesized by the body), such as linoleic acids (from which arachidonic acid derives) and linolenic.

In a balanced and healthy diet it is important to limit the consumption of saturated and hydrogenated fats, as they entail an increased cardiovascular risk and prefer, instead, unsaturated fats such as those represented by extra virgin olive oil and those present in fish or oil seeds.

The recommended daily intake varies from 25 % to 35 % of total daily calories. Olive oil contains monounsaturated fats and a whole series of other nutrients such as polyphenols with antioxidant function, vitamin E and anticancer compounds: olive oil is the main food of the Mediterranean diet and must never be missed on your dishes.

Blue fish (salmon, tuna, mackerel, sardines) contains polyunsaturated fats of the omega 3 series. These fats are called essential, because the human body is not able to synthesize them and must be introduced from the outside with food. In recent years, numerous studies have highlighted the vital importance of these lipids, as they have many beneficial effects on our health and even in the prevention of many diseases (premature aging, heart attacks, depression, Alzheimer's, senile dementia, etc.).

Oilseeds are valuable and very useful foods to eat as they contain fat-soluble vitamins, minerals such as magnesium and polyunsaturated essential fats similar to those contained in fish. Almonds, walnuts, hazelnuts, linseed, pumpkin seeds, sunflower seeds, sesame seeds, pistachios, cashews, etc. can be inserted in the daily diet by adding them, for example, to salads or consumed at breakfast or in the snack.

Hydrogenated and trans fats, contained for example in vegetable margarine and in some oils such as rapeseed oil, are to be avoided. In fact, they are harmful to cell membranes and increase LDL cholesterol, blocking even some mitochondrial breathing processes. Unfortunately, these fats are very present in baked and packaged products, so it is important to always read the labels and check their absence.

Chapter 8 - Vitamins

Vitamins, essential organic compounds in many vital processes, are not synthesized by the body, so it is necessary to integrate them through nutrition. The amounts needed are very small (some milligrams or micrograms per day) and for this reason they are considered micronutrients, in contrast to macronutrients (carbohydrates, fats and proteins) that should be taken in much larger amounts, or tens or hundreds of grams a day. Vitamins are divided into fat-soluble and water-soluble vitamins, based on their solubility in fat and water.

Fat-soluble vitamins

Vitamin A refers to a series of compounds that in nature are found in different forms: retinol and retinal acid. Plant precursors of vitamin A are carotenoids, mainly beta-carotene. This vitamin is essential for cell differentiation, foetal development, immune system, skin and vision. Its deficiency causes mainly night blindness, dryness of the cornea and opacization and corneal ulcerations, while its excess induces fetal malformations, liver damage and, in the case of ingestions of very high quantities, cerebral edema and coma. The recommended daily dose corresponds to 6-700 µg. It is contained in milk, butter, cheese, eggs and, in general, in foods containing animal fats. Carotenoids and beta-carotene are present in colored vegetables.

Vitamin D exists in two forms: cholecalciferol, or vitamin D3, and ergocalciferol, or vitamin D2. Cholecalciferol is mainly synthesized by the body and is formed in the skin by the effect of sunlight; ergocalciferol is taken with food. Both of these forms require activation by the kidney and liver that transform them into 25-hydroxy-vitamin D. In this form, vitamin D promotes intestinal calcium absorption, renal phosphorus elimination and the release of calcium from the bone. Vitamin D deficiency causes osteomalacia, a condition in which the mineral component of the bone is reduced with consequent fractures caused by even minimal trauma. Psychological symptoms such as depression and neurological symptoms such as neuromyopathy may be associated. Under normal renal function conditions, the dosage of 25-hydroxy-vitamin D is a good indicator of its state. Vitamin D deficiencies may be due to reduced dietary intake, poor exposure to sunlight, malabsorption (intestinal diseases), kidney and liver failure. The best food sources are milk and its derivatives. The daily intake recommended by Larns (recommended nutrient levels) is dependent on solar exposure. During pregnancy and lactation 10 μg per day are recommended.

Vitamin E includes 8 compounds, 4 belonging to the class of tocopherols and 4 to that of tocotrienols. It is mainly found in vegetable oils, fruits and oilseeds and the daily recommended amount depends on the amount of unsaturated fat intake. The main biological activity of vitamin E is the antioxidant one, which mainly occurs in lipid environments, such as cell membranes and lipoproteins, where there is a need to defend from oxidation the double bonds of unsaturated fatty acids. Deficiency symptoms are extremely rare and manifest with peripheral neuropathy, altered coordination of movements, myopathy and retinopathy. The determination of plasma levels of vitamin E is a good indicator of the adequacy of its intake.

Vitamin K includes a series of compounds belonging to two families: phylloquinone, substances present in the plant kingdom, and menaquinones, produced in the intestine by the bacterial flora. Vitamin K is essential for the synthesis of certain coagulation factors by the liver. Recently, it has been shown its role also in the metabolism of the bone. Vitamin K deficiency leads to a blood clotting deficit with reduced prothrombin time.

Women over 50 are considered adequate contributions between 60 and 80 µg per day. Vitamin K is contained in vegetables, especially in broad-leaved green plants and in the liver.

Water-soluble vitamins

Thiamine, in the form of thiamine pyrophosphate, plays a key role in the metabolism of carbohydrates and branched-chain amino acids. In its absence, glucose is only partially metabolized, resulting in the formation of excess lactic acid. Deficiency of this vitamin causes heart failure, peripheral neuropathy, coma and intellectual and memory impairments. Minor deficits can result in weakness, reduced appetite, and psychological changes. The requirement is about 1-1.2 milligrams per day (0.5 mg per 1000 kcal introduced). In conditions where metabolic activity increases, such as exercise, pregnancy, and certain diseases, the body needs more vitamin B1. Its dosage in the blood is technically complex and is not performed routinely. It is found in food of animal origin (meat, milk and dairy products, eggs), legumes, whole grains and yeast.

Also called riboflavin, vitamin B2 is a substance that becomes part of enzymes involved in energy metabolism. Its deficiency manifests with lesions in the corners of the lips, glossitis and seborrheic dermatitis. The requirement is 1.3-1.6 mg per day. It is present in numerous foods, such as meat, dairy products, eggs, legumes, whole grains, yeast, vegetables.

Niacin can be synthesized by the body from a protein amino acid, tryptophan. Niacin deficiency gives rise to pellagra: the name given to this vitamin, PP or Pellagra Preventing, is to indicate its effectiveness in preventing this disease, which initially manifests itself with skin lesions, then with intestinal disorders (diarrhea) and finally dementia. The recommended daily intake is 14-18 mg. It is mainly found in meats, dairy products, eggs, legumes, whole grains and yeast.

Pyridoxine is a vitamin mainly involved in amino acid metabolism. Its deficiency causes seborrheic dermatitis and microcytic anemia due to reduced synthesis of hemoglobin. The recommended intake is 1.1-1.5 mg per day. It is mainly found in meat, dairy products, eggs, legumes, whole grains and yeast.

Vitamin B12 is involved in many processes, including the synthesis of nucleic acids and the metabolism of amino acids. To be absorbed at the intestinal level, it must bind with the intrinsic factor, a substance produced by the stomach that has the task to protect it in its path from the stomach bottom to the blood flow. Some gastric diseases, as well as surgical removal of the stomach, cause vitamin B12 deficiency. This deficiency manifests with an anemia characterized by increased red blood cell size, increased plasma levels of homocysteine, atrophy of the lingual papillae, glossitis, neurological damage with disorders of coordination and motor skills, even irreversible. Vitamin B12 can be easily measured in the blood. The recommended daily intake is 2 μg. It is made exclusively from animal sources, so vegan diets easily expose its deficiency.

Folates are a group of substances characterized by a chemical structure similar to that of folic acid; some of their functions are similar to those of vitamin B12. They also fall into enzymatic complexes involved in the metabolism of nucleic acids and amino acids. Deficiency occurs with megaloblastic anemia and increased plasma levels of homocysteine. The dose of folate in plasma is a commonly performed survey and is a good indicator of the state of this vitamin. The recommended daily quantity is 200 μg (400 μg in pregnancy). Good sources of folate are fresh vegetables.

Vitamin C consists of ascorbic acids and hydrocarbons. Its function is complex, intervening in redox reactions, in the synthesis of collagen (the most important structural protein of our organism), in the antioxidant activity in the aqueous phase, in the regeneration of vitamin E and glutathione (antioxidant endogenous substance) oxidized. Vitamin C deficiency causes scurvy, a disease characterized by vascular fragility with gingival bleeding, joint bleeding, petechiae (skin spots due to the breaking of small vessels), susceptibility to infection, weakness and apathy. Vitamin C can be measured in plasma, as an index of recent intakes, and in leukocytes, as an index of reserves. It is recommended to take 60 mg per day. It is found mainly in fresh vegetables and large quantities are contained in citrus fruits and kiwis.

Biotin is a vitamin involved in energy metabolism, as a component of mitochondrial enzymes. Its deficiency, rarely observable, manifests with dermatitis, conjunctivitis and alopecia. It is believed that the necessary doses are between 30 and 100 µg per day. Biotin is made from many animal and plant foods and is also synthesized from intestinal bacterial flora.

Chapter 9 - The Secret Formula to Lose Weight

We assume that to lose weight there are no secrets, or miracle diets, or miracle professionals, but there are methods that can be applied differently according to lifestyle and your energy needs. It is also important that constancy and time are our friends. Beyond the type of diet that can be more or less effective, you have to have patience in losing weight. You will see that by losing just 4 lbs you will feel much more deflated and you will be stimulated to continue in the nutritional path.

Caloric Deficit

To understand the meaning of calorie deficit we must first understand the difference between caloric needs and caloric income. The caloric requirement is the energy that our body needs to support all our physiological functions, basal metabolism, physical activities and daily activities. Theoretically, if we consume as many calories as our caloric requirements, we remain constant with weight. At a time when

71

our caloric intake is greater than our energy needs, we increase in weight. On the contrary, if we consume less calories than our energy needs we will create a calorie deficit and therefore lose weight.

All this, however, is not a perfect mathematical equation, as there are mechanisms that tend to adapt the metabolism when we eat more or eat less. This means that when we take a calorie surplus, a part of it is turned into heat, while when we create a calorie deficit not all the deficit will be turned into weight loss, but the metabolism will adapt to the daily calorie restriction. These are the reasons why we don't get fat or lose weight forever. In fact, our organism has mechanisms of adaptation so that it does not succumb to hunger in the short and medium term. Of course, a calorie deficit that lasts for life as well as a calorie excess that lasts for life will lead on the one hand to malnutrition and then to death, on the other to metabolic diseases and over time to death for cardiovascular diseases.

How to calculate your calorie deficit

To calculate your calorie deficit and therefore know how many calories you have to eat to lose weight, you have to know your starting point, that is, you have to know your current daily calorie intake. To do this you must write down everything you eat daily for at least five days, in which at least one of these must be a holiday day where you will eat more than normal. To know the calories consumed daily, you can make use of some well-made and easy to use applications. The most used are Myfitnesspal and Yazio. First, before you start your food diary, weigh yourself and then write down everything you bring to your mouth. Once you know the calories you consume in these five days you'll have to average them. The value obtained is most likely your daily calorie intake.

Many women when they write down everything they eat tend to self-regulate. The consequence of self-regulation is that they will tend to eat less than they previously ate because of the awareness they acquire about their diet. So if you weigh yourself after five days of a food diary, and you've had a slight weight loss, add an extra 5% to your average. This percentage gap is probably what made you lose weight.

How to go in calorie deficit

Once you get the value with your application, you have to figure out how to go into a calorie deficit. The method consists in eliminating enough calories to allow weight loss to happen.

Suppose you have a daily caloric intake of 2200kcal. Theoretically to have a weight loss of 500 gr per week you will have to eliminate 500 kcal per day from your current calorie income. Therefore, if you want to lose 500 gr per week you will have to eat 1700kcal per day. Our experience tells us that this calorie cut is relatively sustainable.

In order for the diet to be sustainable and not to allow the metabolism to adapt to the calorie deficit, it must not always be the same, but must change day by day. This means that in a week you will have to eat about 12000 kcal. These calories you can distribute as you want, the important thing is that at the end of the week you will have eaten 12000 kcal. For example, from Monday to Saturday you can eat 1500 kcal and on Sunday 3000 kcal. Of course don't weigh yourself the next Monday as you might have a little more water retention. Wait for next Wednesday. Alternatively you could also do a day of 1500 kcal and a day of 1900 kcal. Basically you can manage the diet however you want, the important thing is that it is from 12 thousand kcal weekly.

This method helps you to follow a more conscious and flexible and less rigid intermittent fasting protocol.

How to build the diet based on the caloric deficit obtained

To build your diet based on the calorie deficit you calculated, with the same application you used to make your food diary, you can build your diet based on your work needs, your schedule and your food tastes. From these choices, however, you will have to have some basic rules, otherwise you will tend to always eat the same foods or the one you prefer. Remember that a diet should also be a healthy food lifestyle that helps you change your wrong habits. Therefore try to eat legumes at least twice a week in the absence of an irritable colon, at least twice a week eggs and prefer white meats to red meats and sausages.

If you can't lose weight then you'll probably have to investigate the reasons for your difficulty. A simple method to stimulate your metabolism is to create a calorie deficit for 4 days a week, and then 3 days of normal calorie diet that in the example case would be 4 days of 1700 kcal and 3 days of 2200kcal.

This method will have to be followed for at least 2 months. Of course, in this way, the weight loss will be slower, but necessary to see an improvement in the efficiency of the metabolism. To improve the efficiency of your metabolism you can keep training as well.

There are also some cases in which you still can not lose weight, despite the metabolic stimulus. In this case it is necessary an impedance to identify the metabolic cell mass and in more serious cases it is necessary to do an indirect colorimetry to understand the proper functioning of the metabolism or alternatively hematologic analysis to identify if there are hormonal problems.

<u>Conclusion</u>

We would like to thank you for making it to the end of this intermittent fasting guide. We have done our best to ensure that every information contained is useful and helps you in your journey towards a healthier you.

We know how frustrating it could be to start an intermittent fasting protocol and feeling discouraged by the fact that results do not appear immediately. As we repeated throughout this entire guide, the goal of intermittent fasting is to create a healthy lifestyle that can support you over the years, not just give you a rapid weight loss that is unsustainable over the long run.

By following the intermittent fasting protocols and strategies shared in this book, you will certainly burn fat, lose weight and feel much better. However, as we do not know you in person, our final recommendation can only be the following one.

Before starting an intermittent fasting protocol talk to your doctor and find out whether intermittent fasting could be a good idea for you or not. Remember, never sacrifice your health to fit into that new skirt you just got.

Be healthy and your weight will adapt.

To your success!

Nancy Johnson

Intermittent Fasting

Discover how to Reset your Metabolism with this Weight Loss Guide to Burn Fat, Slow Aging and Live Longer - Detoxify Your Body with these Fasting Strategies and Meal Ideas!

By

Nancy Johnson

work can be in any fashion deemed liable for any hardship or damages that may befall them after undertaking information described herein.

Additionally, the information in the following pages is intended only for informational purposes and should thus be thought of as universal. As befitting its nature, it is presented without assurance regarding its prolonged validity or interim quality. Trademarks that are mentioned are done without written consent and can in no way be considered an endorsement from the trademark holder.

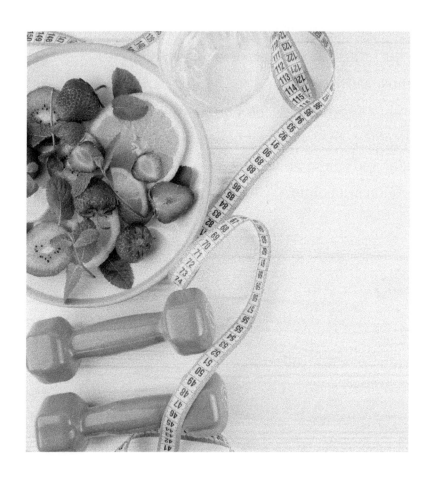

Table of Contents

Introduction

Most women over 50 feel as if they have lost their ability to be attractive, healthy and feel good in their own bodies. This is due to the fact that in today's world, we are spending more and more time at home and we have significantly reduced our need for food. However, even if we do not need as many calories as we did in the past, most of us are still eating as if they were running a marathon a day.

Therefore, it should not come as a surprise that most women over 50 are out of shape, overweight and unhealthy. Thanks to researches and scientific studies conducted by incredible nutritionists, it is now possible to overcome the negative effect of a sedentary life. In fact, intermittent fasting seems like the perfect solution for all those women that want to burn fat, lose weight and gain a healthy and new lifestyle.

The need of all these women is what inspired the writing of this book. In fact, in the next chapters you are not going to find complicated explanations of scientific topics that, even if interesting, do not give you a clear direction on what you can do to start feeling better. On the contrary, while writing this book, a great effort was made to make sure that each concept is followed by a subsequent strategy that can be implemented in a healthy intermittent fasting protocol.

By reading this book you will get all the information and practical steps you need to follow to start intermittent fasting in just a few days. We advise you to talk to your doctor before changing your diet as intermittent fasting is not suitable if you have certain healthy conditions.

Please, be aware that the goal of this book is to give you accurate information on intermittent fasting, but it does not take the place of a professional opinion. We hope that you can find motivational and informative insights that help you make a change for the better.

To your success!

Nancy Johnson

Weight Loss for Beginners

Chapter 1 - An Introduction to Fasting

Before beginning our discussion about intermittent fasting, it is important to have a good understanding of what fasting actually is in a more general sense. In the next few pages we are going to lay out the basics for the rest of the book, so pay close to attention.

Although cases of prolonged fasting due to lack of food are extremely rare in our society, voluntary food deprivation is often undertaken for political, social or religious reasons. Since humans can survive absolute fasting for about 24-30 days, the body's physiological response to this deprivation can be divided into 4 phases, respectively called the post-absorption period, short fasting, medium fasting and prolonged fasting. Let's take a look at them one by one to understand them better.

Post-absorption period

It occurs a few hours after the last food intake, as soon as the foods introduced in the last meal have been completely absorbed by the intestine. On average it lasts three or four hours, followed, under normal conditions, by an ingestion of food that breaks the temporary state of fasting.

In the post-absorption period there is a progressive accentuation of hepatic glycogenolysis ("breakdown" of glycogen into the individual glucose units that make it up), which is necessary to cope with the glycemic drop and supply extrahepatic tissues with glucose.

Short-term fasting

In the first 24 hours of food deprivation, metabolism is supported by the oxidation of triglycerides and glucose deposited in the liver in the form of glycogen. Over time, given the modest amount of hepatic glycogen stores, most of the tissues (muscle, heart, kidney, etc.) adapt to use mainly fatty acids, saving glucose. The latter will be destined above all to the brain and anaerobic tissues such as red blood cells which, in order to "survive", absolutely need glucose. In fact, they cannot use fatty acids for energy purposes. Under similar conditions, the cerebral demands for glucose amount to 4 g/hour, while those of the anaerobic tissues amount to 1.5 g/hour. Since the liver cannot obtain more than 3g of glucose per hour from glycogenolysis, it is forced to activate an "emergency" metabolic pathway, called gluconeogenesis. This process consists in the production of glucose starting from amino acids.

Fasting of medium duration

If food deprivation lasts beyond 24 hours, the action described in the adaptation phase continues with a progressive accentuation of gluconeogenesis. The amino acids necessary to satisfy this process derive from the breakdown of muscle proteins. Since there are no protein deposits in the body to be used for energy purposes, the body, in order to survive the fast, is forced to "cannibalize" its muscles. This process is accompanied by an inevitable reduction in muscle mass, with the consequent appearance of weakness and apathy.

In the early stages, gluconeogenesis is capable of producing over 100g of glucose per day, but soon enough the efficiency of this process decreases to around 75 g/day. Unlike what happens during the first phase, this quantity is no longer sufficient to ensure an adequate supply of glucose to the brain. Therefore, this organ is forced to increasingly resort to ketone bodies, three water-soluble molecules deriving from the oxidation of fats in conditions of glucose deficiency. The overproduction of ketone bodies (a process called ketosis), while prolonging the survival of the organism by a few days, causes an important increase in blood acidity.

During fasting periods of medium duration, which extends up to the twenty-fourth day of food deprivation, the recourse of other tissues to lipid oxidation increases more and more, with a general view of maximum saving of blood glucose.

Prolonged fasting and death

This phase begins when the fast lasts beyond the 24th day. The body has now exploited all the protein resources, including plasma proteins. The mix of ketosis, the lowering of the immune defenses, the dehydration and the reduced respiratory efficiency (given by the catabolism of the proteins of the diaphragm and intercostal muscles) condemns the individual to an unfortunate fate.

So should you be afraid of fasting? That's a reasonable question and if you bought this book is because you are interested in seeing what it can do to help you lose weight. Let's be clear from the start: no, fasting is a great solution to burn fat and get healthier. However, there are some important things to point out to avoid making bad mistakes that can result in health damages.

Many people resort to fasting driven by fashions, advertising or food and health beliefs that are at least questionable. Voluntary abstinence from food intake is understood, in these cases, as a moment of physical purification, aimed at eliminating toxins accumulated due to an incorrect diet.

To analyze this fact, after having broadly described the biochemical aspects, we can start from two assumptions. The first, irrefutable, is that we have plenty of food available, a high-calorie food that is often the basis of obesity; in short, we eat too much and the consequences are there for everyone to see. In fact, overeating and a sedentary lifestyle are among the very first causes of death in industrialized countries, including the US. The second point is that a moderately low-calorie diet, summarized in the Japanese saying "hara hachi bu" (get up from the table with an 80% full stomach), is one of the best strategies for living longer and healthier.

While many people should cut down on their food intake, there is no need to resort to extreme solutions such as prohibitive diets or fasting. Instead, it is enough, as our grandparents used to say, to get up from the table when you are still a little hungry and keep in mind that a little exercise never hurts.

Fasting, similar to physical activity, is a stress for the body. The difference is that, while sport leads to an improvement in organic abilities, fasting moves in the opposite direction. The lack and prolonged intake of nutrients reduces muscle mass and basal metabolism (up to 40% in extreme cases). Furthermore, the mind becomes cloudy and a global state of debilitation arises, characterized by a decrease in muscle strength and ability to concentrate. All this has nothing therapeutic or detoxifying.

Partial or attenuated fasting, on the other hand, could have positive implications, as long as it is applied rationally. After a Christmas dinner, for example, it is useful to follow a low-calorie diet rich in liquids and vegetables for two or three days. The important thing is to associate these foods with a certain amount of proteins, perhaps obtained from lean fish (which is usually easy to digest), and fats, for example by consuming a handful of dried fruit. In this way you avoid "cannibalizing your muscles" and depressing your metabolism excessively and then paying the consequences. This last point must also be clear to those who resort to fasting in extremis to lose weight before summer. In fact, a few pounds can be lost but the amount of energy associated with each unit of weight lost is very low. In other words, weight loss is mainly linked to increased diuresis and muscle catabolism induced by prolonged fasting.

As you might have noticed, even if this book is about intermittent fasting for weight loss, we are not advocating the use of fasting without pointing out the importance of doing things the proper way. In fact, the main reason we decided to write this book is to share the right information that can actually make a difference when starting out with intermittent fasting. Your health is extremely important and we would never advise you to do extreme things just to lose a few pounds.

Now that we are done with this disclaimer, we can finally focus on how you can use intermittent fasting to start losing fat.

Weight Loss for Beginners

Chapter 2 - Intermittent Fasting and Juicing

Some women might find juicing an interesting way to take intermittent fasting to the next level. While in the long run we feel it is too stressful for the body and the mind, if done for a couple of days every month it can truly help you lose weight and purify your body.

In this chapter we dive a bit deeper into this topic and try to understand how to go about juicing. As you will soon discover, juicing while on an intermittent fasting protocol has some interesting and particular details that should be known before beginning this practice.

A juice-only fast is ideal for ridding the body of toxins and promoting weight loss. Plus, it's a healthier type of detox than simple water-based fasting, especially for those who aren't used to it. In fact, the body still receives large amounts of vitamins and nutrients. This chapter will teach you to follow fasting safely and effectively, but you should definitely talk to your doctor about fasting before embarking on it.

Set a goal

Those women who are already experienced with fasting can choose a juice-based diet that lasts approximately 3 weeks. However, if this is your first time, it is recommended to start with a smaller, more manageable goal, such as three days. Fasting can be difficult, both physically and mentally, so it may be easier to start with a reachable goal. It is better to successfully complete a short fast than to falter in the middle of a long one.

A 3-day fast is actually an integral part of a program that lasts 5 days. In fact, you have to calculate 24 hours to get the body accustomed to fasting and another 24 to return to your usual eating habits.
If this is your first fast, it may be helpful to convince a friend to go through the process together. You can motivate each other, and a bit of competitiveness will keep you from giving in to temptation.

Go shopping at the supermarket

For a juice fast, you need large amounts of fresh fruits and vegetables, probably more than you think. It is very important to buy organic agricultural products, not treated with pesticides. The idea of doing such a diet is to get rid of the toxins you have in your body, not introduce any more.

Fill up on oranges, lemons, limes, tomatoes, spinach, kale, celery, carrots, cucumbers, apples, grapes, blueberries, beets, garlic and ginger root.

If possible, you should also get good quality spring water, bottled by a company that uses food-grade plastic or glass containers. Drinking lots of water is an integral part of the diet.

Invest in a good juicer

Having a quality juicer is essential to performing this fast, since it maximizes the amount of juice you get from fruits and vegetables, and saves you time and effort in preparation and cleaning. Make sure the juicer has a power of at least 700 watts, so that it can effectively squeeze any type of fresh fruit you introduce. You should also look for a juicer that has as few parts as possible to assemble and disassemble, as this will speed up the process.

Buying a new juicer can be a considerable expense, but the investment is worth it, especially if you plan to do this fast regularly, integrating it into your lifestyle. Generally, you have to spend around 200 dollars to buy a good juicer, but it could last you 15-20 years.

It is not possible to replace the juicer with the blender to accomplish this fast. If you use the blender, you will end up with a smoothie, not a juice. A smoothie retains the fiber of fruit and vegetables. While this is usually good, you don't need fiber while doing a juice fast. This is because the body uses too much energy when digesting them, the energy it needs to get rid of toxins.

Decide when to do the juice fast

Timing is an important aspect of every fast. You need to make sure you have enough time in the morning to make juices and don't plan on activities that require a lot of energy while fasting, especially if it's your first time. Remember it lasts 3-5 days. Many people who decide to try this method without ever having done it before plan it over the weekend, from Friday to Sunday, when they can stay at home for long periods of time.

Some suffer from headaches and low vitality when following this path (while others report having higher energy levels than usual). Additionally, you may feel the need to take a mid-afternoon nap to conserve energy.

You should also remember that juice fasting stimulates the elimination of toxins from the body, so the body will need to get rid of waste frequently. For this reason, it is best to stay close to a bathroom while fasting.

Prepare your body for juice fasting
Before the actual fast begins, which will last for 3 days, you need to remember that you need 24 hours to prepare your body for the experience. You can do this by eating only raw fruits and vegetables in the 24 hours before fasting. If you like, you can get your body used to it by drinking only juices for breakfast and lunch, and then prepare a solid dinner of salad or other raw fruit and vegetables.

Some people also recommend clearing the body with a purgative (a natural laxative) or enema before the fast begins, but this is optional and we do not recommend it for beginners.

Make enough fresh juice every morning
If you have enough time when you wake up, you can save yourself a good deal of effort throughout the day by preparing all the juices you will drink during the day. Then, keep them in the refrigerator until you are ready to consume them. Alternatively, you can simply prepare the fruit and vegetables

you intend to use for each juice, and place them in airtight bags in the refrigerator until you can make the juice.

Experiment with different combinations of fruits and vegetables to get tasty and unusual results. Try to think carefully about the flavors that would work well when mixed; in this way, drinking juices will be a pleasure rather than an obligation.

When doing a juice fast, you should try to keep a ratio of 20:80 between fruit-based and vegetable-based juices. Fruit juices actually contain a lot of sugars, which are more difficult for the body to assimilate, so maybe limit their consumption in the morning. For lunch and dinner, on the other hand, prefer vegetable-based juices.

Drink as many juices as you want throughout the day

This juice detox shouldn't make you starve. The body needs the vitamins and nutrients in the juice to keep you active and perform that important task of eliminating toxins. For this reason, there is no limit to the amount of juice you should drink over the course of a day. Whenever you feel hungry or thirsty, drink a smoothie. You should consume at least 4 servings a day. If you have read the previous chapters, you know that this is a big difference if compared to the standard intermittent fasting protocol.

If you want to do your juice-based detox for weight loss, you should still avoid limiting your juice intake. With this fast, the body is already deprived of enough calories; reducing the juice intake will therefore send it into survival mode, and this will lead him to retain more weight. So, stick to a minimum of 4 drinks per day.

Drink lots of water

Keeping yourself hydrated is extremely important during a juice-based fast. In fact, water helps you eliminate toxins from the body, and allows you to regain hydration after the purifying action. Plus, it allows you to keep hunger pangs in check. You should aim to consume at least 500ml of water with each juice; you can either dilute the juice 50% with water or ingest the 2 drinks separately, one after the other. You should also drink additional water in between juices.

Drinking herbal tea is another great way to get more water, as long as you prefer the healthy, theine-free versions.

Do not train too hard

While fasting, a little bit of physical activity allows you to distract your mind from hunger pangs, and will help boost your metabolism. A short walk outdoors or some simple yoga poses are all it takes to stay healthy, but avoid exercises that are more vigorous than these, as they may make you feel weak.

Follow the juicing schedule for the next 48 hours, drinking as much juice and water as you like. If you run out of fresh fruits and vegetables, you need to go back to the supermarket. You should also keep experimenting with different recipes to make the juices varied and interesting.

Don't lose your focus

As enthusiastic as you feel at the start of the purification, you will surely find yourself facing temptations and testing your willpower over the course of these 3 days. You will become more sensitive to smells and solid foods will seem inviting like never before. Stay strong and remember why you decided to start a juice fast in the first place. You are getting rid of harmful substances that have accumulated in the body for so many years and are losing weight at the same time. You will feel much better in the end, both physically and mentally, and appreciate the satisfaction of successfully completing your first juice detox. Some women like the fasting process and claim to experience a net increase in energy instead of a drain. Maybe, you will be one of these lucky women.

Try not to think about fasting by engaging in relaxing and rejuvenating activities, such as meditation, reading, stretching and manual projects. By not having to plan your day between meals, you will have much more free time at your disposal.

Take a day to get your body used to the end of the fast. This day will be similar to the day before the detox: you will only eat salads and fruit. Consume small portions so you don't overload your stomach and digestive system.

Gradually return to normal food consumption

After letting your body get used to it, you can progressively return to your usual diet by introducing foods such as eggs, dairy products, rice and whole grains, lean meats. However, you should try to refrain from consuming processed foods to avoid undermining the good work done during detox.

Eating pizza or other processed foods right after you finish your juice fast is not a good idea, and this could also make you feel sick.

Think about introducing a 24-hour weekly juice fast into your intermittent fasting routine. Detoxifying your body with juices once a week will help you maintain the purifying level you have reached with this experience. In fact, it's pretty simple to implement, because you can divide these 24 hours over 2 days. The night before, start with an early dinner, then eat nothing else for the rest of the evening. Sleep for 8 hours, then drink juice for breakfast and lunch the next day. Finally, you can have a solid meal at dinner time, when the purification is complete-

Next time, try fasting longer

Once you have successfully completed a 3-day juice fast, you can take it one step further to make regular detoxes last longer. If you want, commit to completing a 7 or even 14 day juice fast. As daunting as it may seem, many women who have some experience with intermittent fasting argue that juice fasting actually gets easier when periods without solid food get longer. The body gets used to not feeling hungry on its own, because it recognizes that it is getting all the nutrients it needs from the juices.

Either way, be careful. With longer fasts, the body begins to eliminate toxins through the skin and lungs, and you may find that you have a strange or unpleasant smell.

If you are juice fasting longer, you should include protein and iron supplements in your juices to get more energy and avoid becoming anemic. These supplements are available in drug stores and health food stores.

We highly recommend introducing juice fasting into your regular intermittent fasting protocol. However, if you are just starting out, our advice is not to overdo. If you find yourself struggling to keep a healthy intermittent fasting regimen, stick to that before introducing this variation.

Weight Loss for Beginners

Chapter 3 - Practical Tips to Complete a Fast

In this chapter we are going to discuss some practical tips that will help you complete your fast without feeling overwhelmed by the different feelings and emotions you might experience.

There are many reasons why people choose to fast. Your fast may be designed to make you lose weight or detoxify you, or be part of a spiritual practice. Whatever your reasons, facing and overcoming a fast may not be easy. Don't worry though, with the right preparation, determination and self-care you will be able to reach your goal.

As we have mentioned time and time again, before embarking on a fast, it is always good to consult a doctor. Changing your diet drastically will have a noticeable effect on your body, especially if you have some underlying disease that could get worse with fasting (for example, diabetes). Whatever your health situation is, it is always advisable to consult your doctor before starting a fast.

Many people decide to fast for religious reasons rather than in an attempt to lose weight, detox or regain their physical shape.

However, it should be noted that all religions, including Islam, Catholicism and Judaism, allow an exception to be made for all those whose health does not allow fasting in safe conditions. Nonetheless, we think that if you are reading this it is because you are interested in losing weight, not in following some spiritual or religious practices.

Before starting to fast, hydrate your body properly
Without ingesting food, the human body appears to be able to survive for weeks, or in one documented case even for months, but without water it will quickly collapse. Being made up of about 60% water, in order to function, our organism and each of its cells have a considerable need. Without water, most people would die within three days. As you have learned so far, there are different forms of fasting, but in any case, water should never be completely denied. During the month of Islamic Ramadan, believers are forbidden to drink water for long periods of time, but whatever your form of fasting it is important to prepare your body for a nutritional deficiency by "super-hydrating" it in advance.

During the days leading up to the fast, drink plenty of water on a regular basis. Also, before the last meal before fasting begins, take at least 2 liters of moisturizing fluids.

To avoid the risk of dehydrating the body, also avoid foods that are very salty or high in sugar, such as sweet and savory snacks and fast food.

Limit your caffeine intake

Many of the drinks we consume every day, such as coffee, tea and energy or carbonated drinks, contain large doses of caffeine, a substance capable of changing our mood and causing a real addiction. If you are used to taking caffeine and suddenly cutting it out of your diet, you will most likely experience withdrawal symptoms. When you eat normally, these symptoms can go almost unnoticed, but during a fast, even a short one (even for a single day), the signs of crisis can be strongly felt.

Common symptoms of caffeine withdrawal include headache, fatigue, anxiety, irritability, sadness, and difficulty concentrating.

To avoid these unwanted side effects, work to break the habit early by gradually reducing your caffeine intake in the weeks leading up to the start of the intermittent fasting cycle.

Cut down on smoking

If you are addicted to tobacco, you may have more difficulty than having to do without caffeine. Nonetheless, being able to quit smoking is even more important than giving up caffeine. By smoking on an empty stomach, your body and health will be hit hard and you may feel nauseous and dizzy. Tobacco consumption during an intermittent fasting protocol increases blood pressure, heart rate and lowers the skin temperature of the fingers and toes.

If you are having a hard time quitting smoking, even temporarily, see your doctor for a more effective strategy or read books about it. There are some pretty useful guides out there.

Choose foods that are high in carbohydrates

The term "carbohydrate" itself means "carbon rich in water". Unlike proteins and fats, carbohydrates bind to water and allow the body to stay hydrated for longer periods of time. This quality of carbohydrates is very important when preparing for a fast. During the weeks leading up to it, consume large amounts of carbohydrate-rich foods so your body can keep its water reserves tight. We advise you try some of the following foods before and during your intermittent fasting protocol.

- Bread and pasta prepared with multigrain, wholemeal flours and different types of cereals;
- Starchy vegetables (potatoes);

- Vegetables (lettuce, broccoli, asparagus, carrots);

- Fruits (tomatoes, strawberries, apples, berries, oranges, grapes and bananas).

Keep the mealsize under control

In the days leading up to your fast, you may be tempted to overeat to fill up on vitamins, nutrients, and calories. The basic idea will be to fill up in advance to be able to last as long as possible without eating. In fact, however, ingesting large quantities of food will only accustom your body to large meals and, once you stop eating, you will actually feel even more hungry. It is also advisable to vary the meal times every day so that the body does not get used to receiving food at specific times.

Before starting the fast, have a large meal, but don't binge. After eating high-carb foods for days, many women choose to have a "last" protein-rich meal to feel satisfied for a longer period of time and to enter the fast more easily.

Before your final meal, don't forget to take a substantial amount of moisturizing fluids to facilitate a smooth transition to fasting.

Keep busy

Hunger is a primary feeling related to the whole body and, if left free to do, can take control of the mind. Being obsessed with it is the quickest way to failing to overcome fasting. Distract yourself as much as possible by constantly keeping yourself busy.

Engage in light, enjoyable activities, such as chatting with friends or reading a good book.

Taking care of those chores and tasks that you usually put off is another way to effectively keep yourself busy. When the aim is to be able to distract you from hunger, even the hypothesis of cleaning the whole house may not seem so bad!

When you are following an intermittent fasting protocol, reduce the amount of exercise you do

In some cases, based on the reasons and nature of the fast, more vigorous activities may not be recommended or permitted. If you are doing "intermittent fasting," where you fast regularly for a short period of time every given number of days, you are more likely to lose weight. Training a carbohydrate-deficient body means forcing it to burn fat to sustain itself; for many this could be a primary goal. However, note that, at the same time, your body will also begin to burn proteins and muscle mass. The best thing you can do is exercise at a slow pace and avoid exhaustion with a cardio workout.

If you intend to fast for a long time, avoid very tiring activities. Those who follow intermittent fasting simply abstain from food for short periods of time. Even if you have to avoid cardio training, it is good for them to exercise because they will soon give their bodies new fuel. If you intend to fast for several days, however, it is best to avoid any energy-intensive activities. Otherwise you would otherwise feel much more tired than when you do them by feeding normally. Fasting for an extended period, rather than intermittently, means not providing your body with any fuel for a long time. This is why we always recommend women over 50 years of age to follow an intermittent fasting routine, rather than doing prolonged fasting.

Get enough rest

When you sleep, you think you are calm and relaxed, but in reality your body is working to take care of itself. The night's rest gives it the opportunity to repair muscles, form memories, regulate its growth and appetite through hormones. When you fast, lack of food can cause problems with concentration.

Regular naps throughout the day have been shown to improve alertness, mood, and mental sharpness.

Get your body at least 8 hours of sleep each night and take regular naps throughout the day while on an intermittent fasting protocol.

Hang out with other women who are fasting like you

Those who are fasting for spiritual reasons will be facilitated because many of their friends and acquaintances belonging to the same place of worship will be doing the same. Even if you are fasting for health reasons or to purify yourself, it is still advisable to seek the company of a friend who does the same. Being surrounded by people who are on the same path as you will allow you not to feel alone in this experience. Whatever your goals, commit to motivating and empowering each other to achieve them.

Don't talk about food while on an intermittent fasting protocol

Don't put yourself in uncomfortable situations where you might feel sorry for yourself. Even in the presence of other people like you who are facing a fast, do not allow the conversation to turn on the lack and desire for food. By obsessing over the thought of food you will end up not being able to stop thinking about it and you will risk taking a false step as soon as you find yourself alone. Instead of describing what you are missing, develop your conversations in positive terms, for example by analyzing the many benefits you will derive from this experience. Alternatively, you can talk about something completely different, such as the movie you have just seen or a current situation you are dealing with.

As long as the fast is in progress, avoid accepting any invitation involving a meal, even from friends. Even if they didn't tempt you to break your fast by eating in front of your eyes, they would force you to have a difficult and painful experience.

Describe your intermittent fasting protocol in a journal

Even when you can count on the support of a friend to help you stay responsible, sharing some frustrating moments and feelings may not be easy. A diary will then allow you to keep your thoughts private and give a free space to your emotions. If you want, in the future, you can re-read your words to perform a thorough analysis. You can write in your diary as you normally would, recounting simple daily events, or choose to focus exclusively on fasting-related issues. Either way, many of your intimate thoughts are likely to be related to your intermittent fasting protocol in some way.

Don't censor yourself! Even if you are following an intermittent fasting protocol for religious reasons, do not hold back from expressing your possible desire to end the fast. With the simple act of writing down your thoughts, you will be able to cope with them better and let them escape from your mind, and stop feeling obsessed with them.

Plan to break your fast

However hungry you may be at the end of your fast, it will be important to resist the temptation to binge at the earliest opportunity. During an intermittent fasting protocol, the body implements mechanisms that allow it to adapt to the lack of food by slowing the production of those enzymes that facilitate digestion. By binging immediately after stopping it, you will force your body to handle a quantity of food that it is currently unable to process, putting you at risk of stomach cramps, nausea and vomiting. During the last few days of your intermittent fasting protocol, you will need to develop a plan that will allow you to easily resume a regular diet.

To start reintroducing fluids, start drinking fruit juices and eating fresh fruit

Of course, in case you have continued to drink only juices, drinking more of them will not exactly "break" your fast. For those who have only been drinking water though, drinking and eating high water content juices and fruits is the best way to allow the body to return to normal. As we fast, our stomach tends to shrink in size, therefore, by drinking juices and eating fruit initially, we may be able to feel satisfied quickly.

You can follow the tips discussed in the chapter dedicated to juice fasting to see how to properly reintroduce fluids after a long intermittent fasting protocol.

Facilitates the transition to small solid meals
Instead of preparing a single large meal with which to end your fast, have snacks or small meals spread throughout the day. To avoid prematurely overloading your sleeping digestive system, stop eating at the first signs of satiety. Initially it is good to focus only on foods with a high water content such as the following.

- Soups and broths
- Vegetables
- Raw fruit
- Yogurt

Chew your food carefully

When breaking a fast, chewing has two main tasks. First, it prevents you from eating the meal too fast, and in this regard it is good to note that the brain takes about 20 minutes to process the information it receives from the stomach and realize that this organ is full. Eating too quickly leads to binge eating, which is dangerous when coming out of an intermittent fasting protocol. The second benefit of proper chewing is the breaking down of food into smaller, more easily digestible pieces.

Make an effort to chew each bite about 15 times.

Drink a glass of water before your meal and sip another while you eat to slow down the rate of ingestion. Take a quick sip between bites.

Take probiotics

Probiotics are "good bacteria" that spread naturally in the mouth, intestines and vagina. They promote efficient digestion and are therefore valid allies when we break an intermittent fasting protocol. Choose those foods that contain active lactobacillus cultures, including yogurt, sauerkraut, and miso.

Alternatively, you can help your digestion by taking a probiotic supplement in capsule, tablet or powder form.

Listen to your body

Whatever information you read in this book about the best way to break an intermittent fasting protocol, your own body will let you know what it feels ready for. If after reintroducing fruit and vegetables you feel stomach cramps or feel the need to vomit, don't force yourself any further! Go back to eating only fruit and drinking only juice for another meal, or for a whole day. Allow your body to progress at its own pace. Soon you will be able to digest even a heavier meal or heavier foods again without suffering from any side effects.

Nancy Johnson

Chapter 4 - Intermittent Fasting and Sleep

When starting an intermittent fasting protocol, some women might see a negative reaction in their sleep pattern. It is absolutely normal, but we understand how it can affect your mood and overall ability to keep on going with your fasting when things get difficult.

There are a couple of tips and tricks that you can implement that can assure you are well rested even during an intense intermittent fasting protocol. This chapter is going to dive deeper into this topic and tell you everything you need to know to make the most out of your sleep.

When your sleep is constantly interrupted or you just can't fall asleep easily, it can happen that you are severely tempted to resort to sleeping pills. Still, sleeping pills don't prepare you to sleep properly without them, and they tend to leave many women over 50 tired in the morning, as well as addicted to heavy and prolonged intake of these pills. They are more like a shortcut unable to produce any change, especially in the way we eat.

So, can you sleep without sleeping pills? There are many solutions involving food (and drinks) that can be used to sleep better. Here's how to be generous with your belly so it leaves you alone when you want to sleep.

Find out about the foods and drinks that may make it worse for you to fall asleep
Before choosing foods and drinks that can help you sleep better, it is vital to remove food sources that may be preventing you from falling asleep or sleeping as you would like. The worst are caffeine, alcohol and sugar. The following foods need to be slathered into your diet so you don't deprive yourself of sleep.

- **Caffeine**. Caffeine is present in coffee, tea, chocolate, cola, certain energy drinks and derived foods and medicines. The amount of caffeine in each element varies based on the strength and type of food. In general, it is best to stop drinking or consuming caffeinated products at least five hours before bedtime. The older you are, the more sensitive you are to caffeine, which is able to remove sleepiness, make you stay awake longer than necessary, bring fatigue, heartburn, tremors, etc., and can end up depriving you of deep restorative sleep.

- **Alcohol**. Although alcohol can make you feel sleepy initially, it upsets your sleep while you sleep! Alcohol can reduce REM sleep and the duration of sleep, as well as lead you to sleep more superficially and wake up often during the night. And for beauty lovers, alcohol causes noticeable bags under the eyes!

- **Sugar**. Sugar is found in a broad spectrum of processed, natural and cooked foods. Any form of sugar can interrupt sleep if you take too much. The problem with sugar is the spike in blood sugar it creates, followed by its subsequent collapse; the frequency of this process reduces our energy levels and leaves us fatigued; our night cycles are also disturbed by the low energy level caused by an excessive amount of sugar.

Avoid hard-to-digest foods

What causes indigestion in one person may easily not produce the same effect in another. The point is to know the causes of indigestion and manage them. Some of the more common causes are the following.

- Any food you are intolerant to (those you are allergic to should not be consumed at all) - the most common intolerances are gluten, dairy, chocolate or sugar;

- Large meals before bed. When you don't give your body enough time to break down food and lie down immediately after eating, indigestion symptoms are likely to arise. Stop eating calorie dense foods at least five hours before going to bed. A light and healthy diet not only takes care of weight but also reduces the risk of sleep apnea.

- Onions, beans and peppers can cause indigestion in vulnerable people.

Choose foods that stabilize your energy when following an intermittent fasting protocol

These are foods that allow you to avoid extreme levels of blood suger, while still providing you with the energy you need during the day. Normal energy levels avoid irritability, fatigue, stress and exhaustion; they also improve mood and facilitate sleep making you feel more calm, rested and balanced. Foods that stabilize energy levels include the following.

- Foods rich in proteins: lean meats, cheeses, natural yogurt, eggs, fish, wholemeal bread, dried legumes, beans, lentils, nuts, seeds, etc. they are stable sources of protein that give you energy.

- Chromium-rich foods: Chromium will help your body overcome low sugar levels. It can be found in shellfish, cooked beans and cheese.

- Fresh fruit: it is better than snacks. By consuming it, you will have the benefit of fiber, nutrients and a slow energy release, so avoid replacing it with juices, nuts or desserts. Apples and pears relax the digestive system the most, especially while following an intermittent fasting protocol.

Drink lots of water

Water gives life and is devoid of substances that waste energy. In addition, it provides an important aid to good digestion. Try to drink two liters of water (about eight glasses) a day.

Increase the intake of foods high in tryptophan

Tryptophan helps synthesize proteins, being an amino acid and an essential chemical element. It is found in meat, fish, vegetables and eggs, and its consumption in the hours preceding sleep will release melatonin and serotonin, which can promote sleep. It increases the feeling of sleepiness, lowers the level of spontaneous nocturnal awakenings and helps to increase the amount of restful sleep.

It is recommended to have a main meal about four hours before bed, making sure it has complex carbohydrates and foods rich in tryptophan. Of course, have a meal in the evening only if it is prescribed by your intermittent fasting protocol.

If you are hungry before going to sleep, choose a snack high in tryptophan, but make sure you spend at least an hour between meals and sleep, to allow for adequate digestion.

Some snacks to consider before bed are the following.

- Dried fruit and tofu;
- Cheese and crackers;
- Milk and cereals;
- Apple pie with ice cream;
- Biscuits with cereals and raisins;
- Banana and wholemeal bread toast;
- Bread and peanut butter;

Choose foods with a natural relaxing effect
Calcium and magnesium relax the mind, so foods rich in these elements will increase your chances of sleeping well.

Additionally, there are some foods known for sedative properties like the following.

- Lettuce. It contains a substance linked to opium, as well as atropine, capable of preventing cramps. Lettuce can be drizzled with a pinch of lemon and drunk before bed - much better than sleeping pills!

- Complex carbohydrates. They contain serotonin, which promotes sleep; this category includes pasta, brown rice and oatmeal.

- Mandarin juice. It contains bromine, a relaxing substance.

Pay attention to the glycemic index of foods

As we have mentioned in previous chapters as well, the glycemic index plays an important role while following an intermittent fasting protocol. The GI is a food unit of measurement that refers to the processing speed of the food we ingest. Slower processed food keeps us full for longer and tends to be generally healthier, so it has a low GI. Low GI foods maintain better sugar levels, helping us feel better, more balanced and rested throughout the day. Before bed, a day of low GI foods leaves you naturally tired and ready to sleep. Low GI foods include the following ingredients.

- Wholemeal bread, pasta, rice, sweet potatoes, mixed green salad or lightly sautéed vegetables.
- Dried pulses, lentils, and beans are excellent low GI foods.

The more processed a food is, the higher its GI will be.

Try drinking herbal tea, which is guaranteed to promote sleep. There are many herbs that promote sleep. When transformed into herbal tea via infusion or decoction, they can induce drowsiness. We suggest you drink one of the following types of herbal tea.

- Chamomile: in sachets or home grown and dried. Adding honey or ginger can improve the flavor.
- Verbena: Also known as lemon grass, it helps you sleep.
- Lemon balm: "lemon" member of the mint family, which helps you sleep.
- Passiflora (passion flower): this herb is relaxing. It can be effective against insomnia and anxiety; follow the directions on the package. If you have an irritable stomach, try this tea three times a day.
- Lime: use dried flowers to make tea.

Increase the intake of vitamins and minerals to improve sleep

If you're not already following a healthy intermittent fasting protocol, your nutrient levels may be low. There are many vitamins and minerals important for a good night's sleep, including vitamin B, calcium, magnesium, vitamin C, and chromium.

Taking vitamins and minerals through a healthy diet is always preferable, but sometimes supplements are the only way to get the necessary dose of a specific nutrient; consult a doctor for more in-depth advice.

In some countries it is possible to take melatonin, a hormone considered by some to be a stimulant for sleep during the most intense intermittent fasting protocols. However, take into account the meager scientific evidence about the benefits of melatonin supplements for sleep, and you will inevitably reduce the amount of melatonin your body produces. It is probably best to leave these products to older women, whose melatonin production is physiologically declining.

We understand the importance of sleeping well, especially while on an intermittent fasting protocol. If you follow these tips we are sure you are going to feel much better before going to bed, which is something that will ensure you a good night of deep sleep.

Our advice is to stay away from sleeping pills as much as possible. A healthy intermittent fasting protocol incorporates all the strategic elements needed to sleep well.

<u>Chapter 5 - Intermittent Fasting and Supplements</u>

Supplements play an important role when it comes to following an intermittent fasting protocol in the best possible way. In fact, many women think that it is sufficient to eat good foods when breaking the fast to stay healthy. Research shows that this could not be farther from the truth. In fact, studies have shown time and time again that women that follow an intermittent fasting protocol experience some nutritional deficits even if their diet is on point.

In this chapter, we are going to give you all the information you need to start supplementing your nutrition with healthy products that can help you lose weight, keep it off and be healthy at the same time.

Let's start by giving a clear and simple definition of what food supplements are. Food supplements are products that are used to supplement the normal diet.

Therefore, they are not medicines, although they too are subject to strict regulation by the current legislation.

The food supplements market is extremely broad, it includes products suitable for the most varied needs and containing ingredients of different types. In no case, however, these products can be considered as an alternative to healthy and balanced lifestyle habits and even less as a remedy to stem or repair the damage caused by the incorrect habits mentioned above.

Therefore, the correct approach for the right use of food supplements, involves first of all the knowledge of these products (what are they? What is their purpose?), and secondly the ability of the consumers to understand when they can freely take similar products. Another important thing is to understand when it is necessary to consult a doctor before taking supplements. Although they are not drugs, in fact, even food supplements can give rise to side effects and can have various contraindications. For this reason, in case of doubts and in the presence of pathologies, disorders or particular conditions (for example, menopause), the consultation of the doctor is essential.

Food supplements can be formulated in the form of tablets, effervescent tablets, capsules, gummy candies, powders (in containers with measuring cups, or in single-dose sachets) and solutions (generally, in single-dose vials).

These are free sale products, marketed both in pharmacies and parapharmacies (including online) and in herbalist's shops, supermarkets and other shops, both physical and online.

What are Food Supplements used for?

Food supplements are used to supplement the normal diet in cases where there is a deficit of nutrients, for reduced intake, or for increased needs.

Depending on the type, food supplements can also be used to support diets (for example, adjuvant supplements for low-calorie diets, supplements for vegetarians or vegans) or other treatments, as well as they can be used to support the body's functions in particularly intense or stressful periods (e.g. sports supplements, memory supplements, etc.). In this regard, however, it should be noted that the response to the intake of food supplements may vary from woman to woman; for this reason, it is not possible to say that the intake of food supplements is always useful, in all women and in any situation. Once again, your doctor will tell you if they are a good idea for you.

What do food supplements contain?

The ingredients that can be included in the composition of food supplements are many.

Among these, we recall the following categories.

- **Vitamins**. Vitamins are perhaps the best known ingredients. According to the current legislation regarding these products, the following vitamins may be contained within them: vitamin A; vitamins of group B (B1, B2, niacin, pantothenic acid, B6, folic acid and B12); vitamin C; vitamin D; Vitamin E; vitamin K.

- **Minerals**. They are often associated with vitamins within the well-known dietary supplements of vitamins and minerals. The current regulations provide for the possibility of including the following minerals in the ingredients of these products: calcium; magnesium; iodine; iron; copper; zinc; manganese; sodium; potassium; selenium; chrome; molybdenum; silicon; boron; fluoride and chloride.

- **Amino acids.** Essential and branched amino acids can also be part of the composition of food supplements. Examples of amino acids that can be found in these products are valine, leucine, isoleucine, arginine, carnitine, cysteine, etc. However, please note that, in most cases, the amino acids mentioned above are found in the form of salts or derivatives and not in pure form.

- **Omega series fatty acids.** These are essential fatty acids. Food supplements contain mainly fatty acids of the omega-3 series in association or not with fatty acids of the omega-6 series. However, the lack of the latter is generally rare, which is why omega-3s are often preferred as supplement ingredients.

- **Prebiotics and probiotics**. They are used to promote and restore the normal balance of the intestinal bacterial flora which can be altered due to stress, taking drugs (antibiotics), etc.

- **Herbs, extracts and other herbal preparation.** The herbs and their derivatives that can be used in food supplements are really huge in number, varying according to the type of product that needs to be created.

To cite a few examples, there are food supplements containing parts, extracts or derivatives of psyllium, ginkgo, blueberry, grape, valerian, ginseng, eleutherococcus, hawthorn, turmeric, ginger, etc.

- **Other active substances not included in the categories we just mentioned.** A well-known example is given by coenzyme Q10, but also by some types of enzymes (for example, bromelain), phytosterols, flavonoids, phospholipids, melatonin, etc.

Other ingredients or excipients

In addition to the substances described above, food supplements contain additional ingredients, also known as excipients. These are substances that are added to the final product for different purposes. Among these, we recall the following.

- **Substances that allow the maintenance of the characteristics of the supplement**. As mentioned, food supplements can be made in the form of tablets, effervescent tablets, tablets, capsules, gummy candies, powders, liquids. To ensure that the supplements maintain shape, consistency, dilution, release of the active substances after ingestion or other chemical-physical characteristics, it is necessary to add particular substances to the formulation. For example, substances are usually added to tablets and capsules that allow them to be kept sufficiently compact in order to avoid crumbling by handling; substances are added to the effervescent tablets which allow them to be dissolved in water with effervescence, in fact; substances capable of maintaining the particular consistency can be added to the gummy candies as well and so on.

- **Dyes**. They are used to give the product a captivating color in order to ensure a better visual appearance. Of course, food dyes are used.

- **Coating agents**. They are used to give the surface of the product a uniform, smooth and sometimes shiny appearance.

- **Flavors**. Used to give the product a pleasant flavor.

- **Preservatives and antioxidants.** Used to ensure optimal conservation and non-degradation of the product.

Side effects

In the vast majority of cases, food supplements are well tolerated and, generally, are not responsible for the onset of particular side effects. However, this occurrence cannot be excluded with absolute certainty and, in some cases, it is still possible to encounter the appearance of undesirable effects. The type and intensity of side effects that could potentially occur can vary depending on several factors, such as the following.

- The type of supplement taken and the type of ingredients it contains;
- The presence of any problems, disorders and diseases affecting different organs and tissues, their type and their degree of severity;
- The frequency of taking food supplements and the amount of product taken (Note: it is important to respect the dosage indicated on the package / package leaflet and any doctor's instructions).

Finally, it should be remembered that even the onset of any allergic reactions in sensitive women cannot be ruled out. These reactions can be triggered both by the active substances and by the excipients contained in food supplements.

Side effects and natural food supplements

Many people are led to believe that taking food supplements based on natural products or extracts (for example, medicinal plants) is completely harmless and safe. However, this belief - in addition to being unfounded - could even prove to be dangerous. In fact, it is very important to specify that "natural" is not synonymous with "safe"; therefore, it is necessary to always pay the utmost caution even in the consumption of natural food supplements, even more so if you are pregnant, breastfeeding or if you suffer from ailments, problems or diseases of any kind. On the other hand, it is also true that the active substances contained in food supplements are present in such quantities that - with correct use and respecting the dosage - they should not cause any harm. Despite this, in the presence of particular conditions - such as, for example, allergies and diseases - even a small amount of a given substance can give rise to serious side effects.

Contraindications of food supplements

The main contraindication to the use of food supplements concerns the presence of known allergies to the active substances and / or to one or more of the excipients (flavors, dyes, preservatives, etc.) contained in the product.

In addition to this, the intake of some food supplements containing certain substances may be contraindicated during menopause, and in the presence of disorders and pathologies.

For example, women with heart or kidney disease should not take food supplements so lightly, as even substances that are considered harmless under normal and healthy conditions - such as, for example, some natural extracts, minerals, trace elements and amino acids - could be harmful and dangerous in the presence of pathological conditions. Clearly, given the large number of supplements in circulation and the equally large variety of ailments and pathologies that can contraindicate their use, it is difficult to estimate a complete and exhaustive list of all possible contraindications. Talk to your doctor before starting an intermittent fasting protocol and you will get more information about the right supplements for you as well.

Correct approach

To be able to approach food supplements correctly, it is first of all necessary to know these products, to know what they are, what they are for, for what purposes they were designed and when it is appropriate to use them. In this regard, it is important to underline the fact that, in general, the use of food supplements is advisable only if there is actually a need for them. A healthy woman, under normal conditions, who has no deficiencies of any kind and who adopts healthy intermittent fasting protocols, normally, should not need to resort to any type of dietary supplement.

At the same time, food supplements cannot be considered as the emergency remedy to be used in case of unregulated intermittent fasting protocols and lifestyles. Not surprisingly, on the packaging of these products there is always the phrase:

"Food supplements are not intended as a substitute for a varied and balanced diet and a correct lifestyle".

Let's take a practical example to better understand this concept. Taking so-called anti-aging food supplements - which are normally rich in antioxidants - to counteract skin damage caused by bad habits (such as, for example, smoking or uncontrolled exposure to UV rays) makes no sense, if in everyday life, the aforementioned wrong behaviors continue to be adopted. On the other hand, even if said habits are corrected, it is not certain that the aforementioned supplements prove to be really effective in improving the skin appearance.

For a correct use of food supplements, it is also important to remember that these products are not drugs and, therefore, are not able to cure any type of ailment or disease.

Rather, if the doctor deems it useful and necessary, in the presence of particular health problems or diseases, he can prescribe the intake of supplements as an extra "treatment" to traditional therapeutic strategies.

Another particularly important point is that concerning posology. The quantity of food supplement taken and the duration of the "treatment" - shown on the package or on the package leaflet or expressly indicated by the doctor - must be strictly respected. Even if the supplements are not medicines, in fact, it is always and in any case necessary to follow the recommended doses.

Summarizing what has been said so far, we could say that the correct approach for the right use of food supplements cannot be separated from the knowledge of the following basic concepts.

- Food supplements are not drugs.

- Food supplements are not an alternative to a balanced diet and correct lifestyle habits.

- The use of food supplements does not improve a pre-existing state of health.

- The non-use of food supplements does not compromise or worsen the health of the individual.

- Food supplements are not dietary products. In other words, they are not products intended for a particular diet.

- The recommended dosage must always be respected.

- In the presence of diseases or other conditions (for example, particular allergies and menopause), it is necessary to seek medical advice before taking food supplements of any kind.

Now that we have discussed the basics concepts regarding supplements, it is time to dive deeper into those that are actually recommended when following an intermittent fasting protocol.

Nancy Johnson

Weight Loss for Beginners

Chapter 6 - Choosing the Right Multivitamin for Your Intermittent Fasting Protocol

There are several reasons why women need to take multivitamins when following an intermittent fasting protocol. They are especially important for those who are in menopause or trying to get pregnant, as they offer additional help in supporting the body during these important events. Other women, on the other hand, have to take them to combat a particular deficiency. However, for most female subjects who are in good health, the best way to get vitamins is to eat a healthy diet, rich in fruits and vegetables.

Check with your doctor to find out if you have vitamin deficiencies

Many women think they are not deficient in vitamins, when in fact it may be insufficient to some extent. Normal blood tests do not detect the presence of these essential nutrients nor can they identify the levels of vitamin D produced by the body. Therefore, it is necessary to undergo more specific investigations to make sure that any deficiencies are discovered. In these cases, your doctor can help you develop a meal plan and possibly recommend the vitamins that suit your needs. Your doctor will likely recommend that you take them in the following cases.

- You typically consume less than 1600 calories per day.

- You follow an intermittent fasting protocol that does not contain sufficient amounts of fruits and vegetables. In this case, you should eat 90-180g of fruit and also add 300-450g of vegetables per day.

- You don't eat two or three servings of fish a week. In this case, your doctor may recommend fish oil supplements.

- You have a fairly heavy menstrual cycle: you may be subject to an iron deficiency.

- You have digestive problems that do not allow you to assimilate a sufficient amount of nutrients, while following a healthy diet.

Tell your doctor if you are a vegetarian or vegan

These eating habits tend to be indicated when you want to keep fat consumption and cholesterol levels low even during times when you are not following an intermittent fasting protocol. They are often associated with a lower risk of heart disease, high blood pressure, obesity and type 2 diabetes. However, it is important to make sure you are getting all the proteins, vitamins and minerals your body needs. If not, you may have deficiciens like the following ones.

- **Iron**. Many vegetarians have lower iron reserves than those who are omnivores. Consult your doctor to find out if your iron levels are low.

- **Vitamin B12**. Vegetarians can get it through the consumption of dairy products and eggs, but vegans must take supplements or eat foods enriched with vitamin B12. Read the nutritional values found on soy and rice milk products, on the packaging of breakfast cereals and meat substitutes.

- **Calcium**. Since meat and dairy products are high in calcium, many vegans are particularly prone to low calcium intake. This mineral is essential for maintaining bone health and avoiding fractures. If you are vegan, try to consume calcium-fortified foods, such as fruit juices, cereals, soy, and rice milk. This information is usually shown on the packaging. Also, you should check with your doctor to find out if you need to take calcium supplements.

- **Vitamin D**. The body produces vitamin D when it is exposed to the sun. However, the quantities it manages to synthesize depend on the use of sunscreen, the time of the day, the period of the year, the latitude and the pigmentation of the skin. Vitamin D is important for bone health. If you are concerned that you are not producing enough, consult your healthcare provider to find out if you should take supplements and eat foods enriched with this nutrient, including cow's milk, rice milk, soy milk, orange juice, cereals and margarine.

- **Zinc**. Soy, legumes, grains, cheese and nuts are excellent plant sources of zinc. If your diet is low in these foods, consult your doctor about possible solutions.

- **Long chain omega-3 fatty acids**. They are necessary to preserve eye health and the proper functioning of the brain. Many people get them by eating fish and eggs. If you don't consume these foods, you can also get them through flaxseed, canola oil, walnuts, soybeans, omega-3 fatty acid-enriched bars, or microalgae supplements. Ask your doctor if you need to assimilate them by consuming supplements.

Consider your age.

Postmenopausal women need to be careful about getting sufficient amounts of calcium and vitamin D to prevent osteoporosis. It is an important recommendation especially for older women who, living alone, run the risk of falling and suffering bone fractures. Female subjects over 50 should take the following amount of minerals.

- **800 IU (international units) of vitamin D per day**. Even exposure to the sun allows the body to produce it. Try to get out of the house and take a walk every day to make sure you get some sunlight.

- **1200 mg of calcium per day**. It is an important mineral that allows you to keep your bones strong and protect them from natural deterioration due to body movements.

Consult your doctor about taking vitamins in the prenatal period

If you are trying to conceive a child, are pregnant or breastfeeding, your doctor will likely recommend that you take a prenatal vitamin supplement. It is not a substitute for healthy nutrition, but it can help the fetus get all the nutrients it needs. These vitamins are specially designed for pregnant or breastfeeding women. You should not take them if you are not yet pregnant or if you are not breastfeeding. Prenatal vitamins typically contain the following ingredients.

- **Folic acid.** If you are trying to conceive or are pregnant, you need 600-800 mcg (micrograms) of folic acid per day. It promotes brain development in the early stages of fetal development. However, an overdose could hinder the detection of a possible vitamin B12 deficiency.

- **Iron**. If you are pregnant, you need about 27 mg (milligrams) of iron per day. If you take too much, you risk getting sick and suffering from constipation, vomiting, diarrhea or even life-threatening consequences.

- **Calcium**. It is a vital mineral for pregnant women because it promotes healthy bone development. Pregnant women should take 1000 mg per day. However, most prenatal vitamins only contain 200-300 mg. This means that you have to supplement the calcium requirement. You can get it by eating vegetables, such as broccoli, spinach, kale, turnips, savoy cabbage. Also consider other foods that contain added calcium, such as soy milk and fruit juices. In excessive amounts, it can increase the risk of kidney stones.

- **Vitamin D**. If you are pregnant, you should be getting sufficient amounts of vitamin D to support the baby's bone health. The Mayo Clinic (a non-profit organization for medical practice and research in the United States) recommends 600 IU (international units) of vitamin D per day. You can reach this amount by exposing yourself to the sun and consuming fish (especially fatty ones like salmon), fruit juices with added vitamin D, milk and eggs.

Ask your doctor if vitamin supplements can interfere with the action of medications

Some vitamins can interact with the way the body metabolizes drugs. If you are on medication, ask your doctor or dietician about vitamin supplements before you start taking them to make sure you are safe. Here's what some supplements do to the body.

- Vitamin D can affect blood glucose and blood pressure, but also interact with birth control pills and drug treatments for HIV, asthma, cancer, heart disease, cholesterol problems, pain relievers and other medications.

- Vitamin B6 can increase the risk of bleeding if it interacts with aspirin or other blood thinners. If you are diabetic, ask your doctor about taking vitamin B6 before taking it, as it can affect the blood sugar level. It can also negatively interact with medications for asthma, cancer, depression, Parkinson's disease, and other conditions.

- Vitamin E can also increase the risk of bleeding when taken in combination with blood thinners. It could also affect the action of drugs against Alzheimer's disease, tuberculosis, cancer, asthma, heart disease, seizures and other diseases.

- Vitamin C can interfere with anticoagulants and affect blood glucose and blood pressure, but also interact with oral birth control pills, HIV medications, acetaminophen, Parkinson's disease medicines, antibiotics, anticancer drugs, aspirin, barbiturates, and other substances.

As you can see, it is important to talk to your doctor before taking any supplement.

Consider a multivitamin
The advantage of multivitamins is that most of them are designed to offer the recommended daily allowance (RDA) of different vitamins and minerals. The RDA should be sufficient - therefore, not contraindicated - for most women in good health.

Look at the labels on the products
You should find a table that tells you what percentage of each individual nutrient is contained in the product based on the RDA. The best proportions provide about 100% of the daily requirement of different vitamins and minerals.
If your doctor thinks it helps, you can buy a multivitamin at a drugstore.

Do not take excessive doses of any particular vitamin
If the label on the package indicates that it provides much more than 100% of the recommended daily allowance, then that is what is known as a megadose. For example, 500% of the RDA of a certain mineral is a megadose. In fact, excessive intake of

some vitamins can be harmful and have the following consequences.

- Too high or too low amounts of vitamin B6 can cause problems to the nervous system.

- It is easier to experience an overdose of fat-soluble vitamins (A, D, E, K) rather than water-soluble vitamins, as the excess is not excreted in the urine. For example, too much vitamin A can increase the risk of hip fracture, while too much vitamin D can promote exorbitant amounts of calcium in the blood and cause vomiting and constipation.

- Excessive iron intake can cause vomiting and liver damage.

- Vitamins and minerals are often added to industrial foods and drinks. If your intermittent fasting protocol favors a large supply of certain vitamins, be aware that you may need to reduce your supplement intake since you are already getting the right amounts of these nutrients.

Don't take expired vitamins

Vitamins can degrade over time. This deterioration is more likely especially if you store them in warm, humid places. If they have expired, it is safer and healthier to buy them again. If you're considering taking certain vitamins that don't have an expiration date, don't take them.

Research the vitamins you are considering

The content of vitamins and supplements available on the market is not subject to strict quality control as is the case with food. This means that it is difficult to know exactly what these pills contain.

Check if the supplements you intend to take are present in the special register made available by the Ministry of Health.

Get adequate amounts of folic acid

Women who are not pregnant need 400 mcg of folic acid, or folate, per day. It is a vitamin belonging to group B, which is important for the nervous system. Excellent sources of folic acid include the following foods.

- Whole grains or grains enriched with folic acid

- Spinach;

- Beans;

- Asparagus;

- Oranges;

- Peanuts.

Eat foods rich in iron

The body better assimilates iron from meat, especially red meat. However, if you are a vegetarian, you can still meet your iron needs by increasing the consumption of foods that are rich in iron, even if they are not of animal origin. Before menopause, women should take 18 mg per day. After menopause, the daily intake drops to 8 mg. Excellent sources of iron include the following foods.

Red meat (lean meat is healthier, because it contains less fat);

- Pork;

- White meat;

- Seafood;

- Beans

- Peas;

- Spinach;

- Raisins and dehydrated apricots;

- Foods that contain added iron, such as cereals, breads, and pasta. On the package you will find written if they have been enriched or not.

Calculate if you are getting enough calcium

After menopause, women's daily calcium requirement increases from 1000 mg to 1200 mg per day. It is important to take it in sufficient quantities to prevent osteoporosis. A calcium deficiency can be avoided by consuming the following foods.

- Milk;

- Yogurt;

- Cheese;

- Broccoli;

- Spinach;

- Kale

- Turnips;

- Cabbage;

- Calcium-enriched soy milk and fruit juices;

- Salmon.

Get sufficient amounts of vitamin B6

It is an essential nutrient for the proper functioning of the nervous system. It is rare to suffer from a deficiency, but it is possible to completely avoid this possibility by consuming these foods.

- Cereals;

- Carrots;

- Peas;

- Spinach;

- Milk;

- Cheese;

- Eggs;

- Fish;

- Flour.

Get out in the sun to take enough vitamin D

When exposing to sunlight, don't forget to use sunscreen to avoid sunburn. The recommended amount for women is 600 IU (international units) per day. For women over 50, on the other hand, an additional intake of 200 IU per day is recommended. It is important because it promotes bone strength when, at a certain age, the risk of bone fractures is higher than in younger women. Vitamin D can also be obtained by consuming the following foods.

- Milk;
- Yogurt;
- Salmon;
- Trout;
- Tuna fish;
- Halibut.

Eat carrots to get vitamin A

This vitamin is important for the visual system, cell growth and proper functioning of the immune system. In adequate quantities, it can also help prevent cancer. You can get it by consuming the following foods.

- Yellow vegetables;
- Liver;
- Kidneys;
- Eggs and dairy products.

Cook with an oil that guarantees a sufficient supply of vitamin E

In addition to eggs, cereals enriched with this vitamin, fruit, spinach, red and white meat and nuts, it is contained in many qualities of oil, including the following ones.

- Corn oil;

- Cottonseed oil;

- Safflower oil;

- Soybean oil;

- Sunflower oil;

- Argan oil;

- Olive oil;

- Wheat germ oil.

Protect the health of the circulatory system with vitamin K

Vitamin K is necessary for the blood because it promotes blood clotting. You can get it in sufficient quantities by eating the following foods.

- Green leafy vegetables

- Meat;

- Dairy product.

Chapter 7 - Vitamin C and Vitamin D: Your Best Friends During Intermittent Fasting

Vitamin C and Vitamin D are two of the most important vitamins to assume during an intermittent fasting protocol. In fact, as we have seen in the previous chapters, vitamins can have a profound impact on the result of an intermittent fasting protocol.

In the next few pages we are diving deeper into this topic, trying to highlight the most important factors that make these two vitamins an incredible asset during your diet.

Vitamin C, also called ascorbic acid, is a water-soluble antioxidant that helps keep infections under control, neutralize free radicals, and promote iron absorption. It also helps produce collagen, which is essential for the health of teeth, organs, bones and blood vessels. Unlike most animals, humans do not have the ability to independently produce vitamin C, so it is necessary to assimilate it every day, constantly. Any food containing at least 10% per serving of the recommended daily intake can be considered a good source of vitamin C. The good news is that vitamin C is found in many healthy foods, so for those looking to increase their consumption, it won't be hard to do so.

Vitamin C is essential for memory, helps prevent cell mutations, premature aging and oxidation of fatty foods, and also strengthens the immune system.

Some believe that vitamin C cures or stops the common cold, but there is no convincing scientific evidence for it. However, by strengthening the immune system, it is possible that vitamin C protects the body from pathogens that cause colds, so it may relieve it and perhaps shorten its duration, but it will hardly prevent it. Please be aware of online scammers that tell you that vitamin C is the solution to every health problem, it is simply not true.

Relationship between diet and vitamin C consumption

Most people should be able to get adequate amounts of vitamin C by following a healthy, nutrient-rich intermittent fasting protocol. If you eat junk food, you are unlikely to get a good dose of vitamin C from your intermittent fasting protocol. However, it is enough to change one's eating habits to increase the assimilation of ascorbic acid.

Since vitamin C neutralizes some food inhibitors, such as phytates (found in whole grains) and tannins (found in tea and coffee), increasing your intake of vitamin C can help optimize nutrition and lead a healthier lifestyle.

Relationship between vitamin C and stress

A vitamin C depletion can cause stress. If the tension is constant, it will soon drain all vitamin C stores. Eating foods rich in ascorbic acid or taking supplements when you feel stressed can have a positive effect on your diet and well-being. If you are aware of what you eat and the micronutrients of each food, you can adjust your intermittent fasting protocol to make sure you are getting enough vitamin C.

Symptoms that tend to characterize a possible vitamin C deficiency

When you have health problems, you should always go to a doctor directly to be on the safe side, but the following symptoms may be associated with a vitamin C deficiency: gums, scarring problems and reduced immune defenses against infections. These symptoms are not necessarily indicative of a vitamin C deficiency, but you can speak to your doctor in case you are concerned.

Acute vitamin C deficiency can cause a condition called scurvy, which occurs when the body cannot produce collagen or absorb iron due to vitamin C deficiency.

Few people in developed countries suffer from severe deficiencies. However, if you exclude vitamin C from your intermittent fasting protocol for about 4 weeks, the deficiency can arise rather quickly.

People at particular risk include the elderly, drug users, alcoholics, individuals with mental illnesses, neglected dependents, individuals suffering from eating disorders such as anorexia or bulimia, smokers (they need more vitamin C to cope with the additional stress exerted on the organism) and individuals who tend to have difficult tastes when it comes to eating fruits and vegetables.

Remember that you need to take vitamin C every day. Vitamin C does not remain in the body, it must be constantly replenished. Eating a certain amount of citrus fruits on a given day only serves to temporarily satisfy the consumption of vitamin C. In fact the next day you will have to renew your supplies. It is estimated that women need a minimum of 45 mg of vitamin C per day. The optimal amounts are 90 mg for men, 75 mg for women and male adolescents, 65 mg for female adolescents. Pregnant or breastfeeding women need 75-120 mg per day.

Usually, if doses of vitamin C that exceed the recommended daily intake are taken, the excesses are expelled. In high doses it is not considered toxic, but it increases iron absorption, which can be a problem for those suffering from hemochromatosis (excessive accumulation of iron in the body). Consequently, if you are already eating a balanced diet, it is not necessary to take vitamin C supplements.

Additionally, overdoing vitamin C can cause abdominal pain, nausea, headaches, fatigue, kidney stones, and diarrhea.

Get enough vitamin C during your meals

This is essential to reap all the benefits. Vitamin C supplements are measured in milligrams. Many foods contain it, so consuming them can help you increase your ascorbic acid intake.

Pineapple contains 16 mg of vitamin C, asparagus 31 mg, raw broccoli 89 mg, dried tomatoes in oil 101 mg, raw parsley 133 mg. Apples are so rich in phytonutrients that a single serving has antioxidant properties equivalent to 1000 mg of vitamin C.

Citrus fruits are a particularly rich source of vitamin C. For example, 230g of grapefruit is enough to meet your daily requirement of vitamin C, while a glass of orange juice is equivalent to 165% of your daily intake of vitamin C. Fresh orange juice or an orange is preferable to a packaged juice. Furthermore, the vitamin C contained in citrus fruits helps fight stress because it lowers the levels of the stress hormone and reduces blood pressure, increases the energy level by promoting iron absorption and provides other essential phytonutrients that work in synergy with the ascorbic acid (some of them improve memory).

Pay attention to the recommended doses of vitamin C we mentioned

Consult the nutrition table prepared by the Health Ministry and look for the recommended doses. You will be surprised to find that it is really easy to vary your intermittent fasting protocol in order to include enough sources of vitamin C.

Pay attention to the shelf life of your vitamin C sources. It is not convenient to store them for a long time, in fact over time they will lose their properties. As a result, try to eat foods that are as fresh as possible rather than leaving them in the refrigerator or pantry. For example, if you leave broccoli in the fridge and then boil it, the vitamin C content will drop considerably, while freshly steamed broccoli has much more.

If possible, grow vegetables indoors, just grow broccoli on the balcony and potatoes in a sack or barrel.

Wash the fruit and vegetables, then let them dry. Store them in an airtight container in the fridge and eat them within a few days. Do not immerse or store them in water, otherwise the vitamin C will dissolve in the liquid. It also disperses in the cooking water.

Fresh foods are the best sources of vitamin C, which is found in most fruits and vegetables. In particular, try to eat foods from the cabbage family, red and green peppers, potatoes, black currants, strawberries, citrus fruits, and tomatoes.

Eat lots of green leafy vegetables [27], including broccoli, kale, Brussels sprouts, and spinach, raw or steamed. Use only a small amount of water to maximize the vitamin content.

Go for a spinach-based salad rather than a lettuce-based one. Raw spinach contains more vitamin C. To fill up on ascorbic acid, enrich your salad with tomatoes, green and red peppers. Vegetables lose micronutrients with cooking.

Incorporate more potatoes into your diet
They are another great source of Vitamin C. You may have heard that Vitamin C is concentrated in the peel, but it is not

ture, although it has other benefits. For example, the peel is rich in fiber. When baking potatoes, be sure to eat the peel as well.

Vitamin B and juices

If you count fruit juice when you calculate your daily vitamin C intake, pay attention. The juice contains a lot of calories, not to mention that it does not have the properties of the actual fruit. To increase your consumption of vitamin C, you should make the juice with the pulp, because vitamin C is better absorbed when combined with bioflavonoids, which are found mainly in the pulp.

Drink some fresh juice

Make it at home or buy frozen concentrates and avoid the packaged juices you find in the fridge. Frozen concentrates have significantly higher doses of vitamin C. In fact, the pasteurization process that characterizes industrially produced juices partially eliminates vitamin C.

Vitamin C and supplements

Take vitamin C supplements in tablet form. There are a number of over-the-counter supplement brands. They have different dosages: you should take the one that best suits your needs. If you are unsure, ask your pharmacist for advice.

Use a topical supplement. Vitamin C preparations for local use are good for the skin. Studies have been carried out to evaluate their rejuvenating effect on mature or wrinkled skin.

Use chewable vitamin C tablets. There are supplements in tablet form that taste amazing. They should be chewed well and then ingested.

Use soluble vitamin C tablets, another product to supplement ascorbic acid which usually tastes pretty good. Let the tablet dissolve completely on your tongue. It is recommended not to eat, drink or smoke during this process. It is quite effective when you feel a bit sick, because vitamin C has a positive effect on energy levels and the immune system.

Now that we have discussed the incredible power of vitamin C, it is time to dive deeper into another great vitamin that you should include in your intermittent fasting protocol. We are talking about vitamin D and the next few pages are going to tell you more about it.

Vitamin D is a nutrient that can prevent several chronic diseases, including some cancers. However, many women lack it because most foods don't contain enough of it. In fact, the richest source of vitamin D is the sun, but being exposed to sunlight for too long is dangerous for the skin. It is not easy to satisfy your daily needs for this nutrient, but thanks to an adequate intermittent fasting protocol, careful exposure to the sun and taking supplements, you can get the benefits of this precious element.

Take supplements

Although it is important for health, this vitamin is not present in sufficient quantities in foods, therefore it is not possible to assimilate an adequate dose simply with a healthy intermittent fasting protocol. While you can look for foods that are particularly rich in it, supplements are an important aspect of improving health and increasing this rare resource. You can find vitamin D supplements in two forms: vitamin D2 (ergocalciferol) and vitamin D3 (cholecalciferol).

Vitamin D3 occurs naturally in fish and is processed by the body when it metabolizes sunlight. It is also believed to be less toxic, in large quantities, than vitamin D2, although it is a more potent form and offers greater health benefits.

Most experts recommend vitamin D3 over D2. Ask your doctor for advice on the dosage and quality of the various brands.

Be sure to take magnesium supplements as well. This other element is needed to absorb vitamin D, but is completely depleted during this process. If you only take vitamin D without supplementing magnesium, you can suffer from a deficiency of that mineral.

Choose vitamin D2 supplements if you are vegan. Vitamin D3 is more complete, but it is of animal origin. Therefore, if you are vegan or vegetarian, you will avoid these types of products, regardless of the health benefits. Vitamin D2, on the other hand, is synthetically produced using molds and does not contain products of animal origin.

Increase your sun exposure while still protecting your skin

Although vitamin D is scarce in foods, it is abundant in sunlight. It is important to find the right balance between too much and too little exposure, because you don't have to risk getting burned. To find a good solution, you can spend 10-20 minutes in the sun twice a week, putting sunscreen only on your face. Alternatively, you can spend 2-3 minutes in the sun several times a week, always putting the protection on your face only. Either way, make sure you don't bathe for an hour after being in the sun. Your body needs some time to absorb the vitamin it has produced.

Be careful not to over-expose yourself to UV rays, as they can cause skin cancer. In the United States, 1.5 million cases are recorded each year. Avoid getting burned in the sun, not so much because of the pain, but because it causes damage to skin cells that can cause abnormal and cancerous growth.

Continue to use sunscreen on any other occasions you expose yourself to the sun. You will likely be able to absorb vitamin D even with sunscreen, but its ability to protect the skin from harmful UV rays also limits the production of vitamin D.

Your skin does not need to tan to be able to absorb vitamin D from the sun.

Learn about the factors that can affect sun-triggered vitamin D production

An important factor is the proximity to the equator. In fact, people who live in this geographic area inevitably have more opportunities to expose themselves to the sun than those who live in areas further north or south. The natural color of the skin also affects the ability to absorb vitamin D; individuals with a lighter skin produce it more quickly than those with a darker skin tone, due to the melanin content.

Even if you can't intervene on these factors, you can still choose the time of day to go outside and get sunlight. It is best to expose yourself during the central hours of the day, rather than early in the morning or in the evening, because at this stage of the day the sun is stronger and the body produces more vitamin D.

Expose as much skin as possible to the sun. During these few minutes that you are purposely in the sun, you should not cover your body with long-sleeved trousers or clothing. The more skin is exposed to the sun, the more vitamin D is synthesized. However, use common sense; if you live in an area where the sun is very strong, by respecting this advice you risk getting burned.

Keep in mind that sun exposure is very high even on a completely cloudy day

The body is able to store vitamin D, so if you stay out in the sun systematically in spring or summer, you will have enough for the whole year.

Eat foods rich in vitamin D

While you can't get enough of this element on a normal intermittent fasting protocol, you can still try to get as much of it from foods as possible. The richest natural source is fish, such as salmon, mackerel, tuna and sardines. If you are brave enough you can also try cod liver oil. Dairy products, egg yolk and cheese also contain small amounts of vitamin D.

Look for fortified products. As awareness of the benefits of vitamin D increases, so does the number of food companies that enrich their products with this vitamin. Read the nutrition information label to find out if a product has been enriched. Among the most common are milk and breakfast cereals.

Limit your caffeine intake

Studies have found that it interferes with vitamin D receptors and inhibits their absorption. Due to its effects on vitamin D, caffeine also negatively affects calcium levels in the body, since one function of vitamin D is to promote its absorption. Avoid drinking too many drinks containing this substance, such as coffee, tea, and other caffeinated sodas.

As you might have understood by now, there is not a single thing you can do to ensure adequate levels of vitamin D. Studies have found that supplements are not as effective a source of nutrients as food, but it is also true that foods do not provide enough vitamin D for optimal health. The only abundant natural source of this nutrient - the sun - is also very dangerous when exposure is excessive and can cause cancer. The best approach to increasing vitamin D levels is to combine all three methods: supplements, sunlight, and nutrition.

Benefits of vitamin D

Many studies have shown that vitamin D is very effective as a means of preventing numerous chronic diseases. In particular, it is able to increase the body's ability to absorb calcium, preventing bone problems such as rickets, osteomalacia (softening of the bones) and osteoporosis. Other research suggests that increasing the intake of vitamin D can lower blood pressure, reduce the chances of heart attack and stroke, develop autoimmune diseases, such as rheumatoid arthritis, and multiple sclerosis.

Dangers of a vitamin D deficiency

It is important to put in place all possible techniques to increase the levels of this vitamin in the body, because its deficiency is related to a number of chronic diseases. Hypovitaminosis D is linked to type 1 diabetes, chronic pain - both muscle and bone -

and several types of cancers, including colon, breast, prostate, ovary, esophagus, and lymphatic system.

About 40-75% of the population is deficient in vitamin D, mainly because this nutrient is not abundant in natural food sources and many people live in areas where it is not possible to get enough exposure to the sun. Increased awareness of the correlation between UV rays and skin cancer has increased the use of sunscreens, which lower the production of vitamin D.

Although 40-75% of the population does not meet their vitamin D needs, there are some categories that are more likely to be deficient in this nutrient. You must be aware of these factors in order to act accordingly and monitor your vitamin D levels.

The risk categories are the following.

- Women suffering from photodermatitis for whom sunlight is toxic;
- Women who rarely go outside;
- Women suffering from heliophobia;
- Malnourished women who develop extreme sensitivity to light;
- Women suffering from malabsorption diseases;

- Those women who wear clothes every day that cover them from head to toe;
- The elderly, whose absorption capacity by the skin is lower;
- Women who stay inside buildings all day, for example those who work in shopping centers;
- Women who follow a very strict intermittent fasting protocol without proper knowledge.

Getting tested for hypovitaminosis

See your doctor for a blood test called a 25 (OH) vitamin D test, or calcidiol. Your doctor will take a blood sample from you which will be analyzed in the laboratory.

If the doctor does not want to prescribe a blood test or you prefer another method, you can buy "do it yourself" tests on the internet. They are not very expensive (around 50 dollars) and can be a valid alternative.

It is not always easy to diagnose vitamin D deficiency, because its symptoms are similar to those of many other conditions. For this reason it is essential to check the levels regularly.

When you collect your calcidiol test results you will be able to understand them and change your intermittent fasting protocol based on them. Usually the value is expressed in ng/ml (nanograms per milliliter) or in nmol/l (nanomoles per liter). This indicates the amount of calcidiol in the blood, which in turn is a good reference for understanding the level of vitamin D.

According to the Endocrine Society, if your values are below 20 ng/mL (50 nmol/L), then you are vitamin D deficient. A result of 21-29 ng/mL (52.5–72.5 nmol/L) indicates some nutrient deficiency, but not a severe deficiency.

If your values fall within a deficiency or deficiency range, then make changes to your diet, get out in the sun and take supplements to increase your vitamin D intake.

Some women are better off when they have an amount of vitamin D that hovers around its recommended maximum levels. Find the amount that makes you feel good and keep it in check with supplements and foods rich in vitamin D.

If you follow these tips, you can be sure you will not have issues related to the deficiency of these two important vitamins. We highly recommend you plan ahead your vitamin intake before starting an intermittent fasting protocol.

Nancy Johnson

Chapter 8 - How to Stop Eating Processed Food

We want to dedicate the last chapter of this book to a very important topic. In fact, every intermittent fasting protocol is deemed to fail if you eat processed and unhealthy foods during your meals.

Most women over 50 are used to eating huge amounts of processed foods and this can have negative consequences when it comes to their health. By following the tips and tricks we share with you in this chapter, you are going to be able to improve the quality of your intermittent fasting protocol and conquer a healthier lifestyle.

Industrially processed foods have a bad reputation. They are very often associated with a high calorie content, with added fats and sugars, they are poor from a nutritional point of view and rich instead of chemicals and preservatives. However, the definition of junk food is currently quite broad and includes many different foods. In general, processed food means any food that has been deliberately processed before being eaten. When trying to reduce their consumption, it is important to consider the level of industrial processing. Highly refined, pre-cooked foods, rich in sugar, flavorings, dyes, preservatives or additives to improve texture are typical examples of the foods you should limit or exclude from your intermittent fasting protocol. By cutting out or cutting down on highly processed foods, you can eat healthier and more nutritious. In the following pages we are going to give you some tips to reduce the consumption of these foods.

Keep track of your meals
When trying to eliminate certain foods or food groups from your intermittent fasting protocol, it can help to keep a journal where you can write down your habits. This way, you will be more aware of what processed foods you are eating, when you eat them, and how often.

Buy a diary or download an application on your smartphone. The ideal would be to write down the meals of a few working days and a few weekends. You may find that you eat differently on weekends than on weekdays, even if following your intermittent fasting protocol with precision.

Many times, people choose industrially processed foods for convenience. They are late for work, do not have time to cook, or have no other choice available when they are hungry. Pay attention to your eating habits: maybe you are always late in the morning and end up buying breakfast at fast food, without even getting out of the car.

It can help you to gradually eliminate industrial foods from your diet. As you rule out certain foods, you can replace them with less processed, more natural foods. By noting on paper what you need to eat, you can visually organize the meals for the whole week.

During your free moments, invest time to write down different meal and snack ideas. These notes can also become the basis for the shopping list.

When drafting your personal intermittent fasting protocol, be sure to take into account the amount of "on the fly" meals you need to eat during the week. By planning them in advance, you will be less tempted to take industrial foods.

Clean up the kitchen

Before re-evaluating your intermittent fasting protocol, think about what you typically buy at the grocery store and what you keep in the kitchen. Look in the refrigerator, freezer and pantry for processed foods, so free yourself from any temptation.

The items you need to check include the following.

- sweets such as ice cream, candies, cookies and snacks;

- potato chips, crackers, or pretzels;

- breakfast cereals, sauces, dressings or marinades;

- meats and cheeses;

- frozen appetizers or pre-cooked meals ready to be heated in the microwave.

These are typically all high in preservatives and high in sodium, something you want to limit while intermittent fasting.

Since almost all foods go through a process, decide which ones you want to eliminate and which ones to keep. For example, canned beans are processed, but they are also an excellent source of fiber and protein. Also, as long as you rinse them and throw away the storage liquid, they are considered low in sodium. This is a food that you should consider keeping in your intermittent fasting protocol.

The other processed foods you can keep are the following.
- canned vegetables with no added salt and low in sodium;

- whole grain foods (such as wholemeal pasta or rice);

- pre-washed and chopped vegetables (like ready-made salads in bags);

- totally natural nut butter.

If you don't feel like throwing away all this food, you can donate it to a charity or eat it in smaller doses until you change your intermittent fasting protocol and eat mostly natural foods.

Tips to avoid processed foods while shopping

When you go to the supermarket, you should forgo all processed snacks. Above all, go along the outermost and perimeter aisles, those in which the most wholemeal and natural foods are usually displayed. Try to choose products that come from these departments: fruit and vegetables, fresh meat and fish counter, shelves of dairy products and eggs.

Generally, the frozen food sector is also located around the perimeter of the supermarket and you can find both highly processed and almost natural foods. As long as the products don't contain too many sauces, toppings, and too many additives, they are still considered an acceptable and nutritious choice.

Be wary of the foods you find in the middle aisles. If you need to buy processed foods, choose only healthy and nutritious ones, such as canned beans, whole grains, and canned vegetables. Also make sure they don't contain too many added ingredients. For example, choose plain pasta instead of pasta with added flavorings or sauces, or low-sodium canned vegetables instead of those rich in seasonings or other flavorings.

If some of your favorite foods are in these aisles and you are tempted to buy them, completely avoid going near these shelves. For example, don't go to the area where the candy and chips are located, so you won't be tempted to put these products in your shopping cart.

Read the labels on all packaged foods. Since food processing can vary greatly, reading the labels gives you more details and accurate information about their process, what has been altered and what has been added.

The list of ingredients allows consumers to know exactly the content of the product. The label shows all the elements present in descending order, starting from the main ingredient to the one with the lowest dosage. In addition, you can check if the product contains additives, preservatives or other flavors.

There are several tips or tricks to help the consumer understand if the level of industrial processing is acceptable. Usually, it is advised not to buy those products that contain elements that are difficult to pronounce or incomprehensible. For example, some processed foods contain substances such as: diacetyl (a flavor of butter) or potassium sorbate (a chemical used to prolong shelf life). If you don't know what it means, you don't buy it.

Keep in mind that if a manufacturer brand has patented a proprietary blend (of ingredients such as spices or flavorings), it must indicate the ingredients, but not always the proportions. If the label shows this type of information, you shouldn't buy the product.

Be aware that some additives can make the product more nutritious. For example, some companies add vitamins or minerals to their foods. Even if these substances are unfamiliar to you, they actually improve the nutritional value of food.

Buy and eat fruits and vegetables. These are highly nutritious foods that contain essential substances, such as vitamins, minerals, fiber and antioxidants. At least half of each meal should consist of fruit or vegetables.

Agricultural products that have undergone minimal industrial treatment and which you should focus on are the following.

- fresh fruits and vegetables such as bananas, apples, tomatoes, aubergines;
- pre-cut and washed products, such as salad in bags or pre-cooked steamed green beans;

From canned foods, choose those low in sodium and with no added salt, prepared without sauces or other condiments.

Avoid over-processed products, such as fruit in syrup or sweetened, frozen or canned vegetables rich in sauces or other condiments.

Buy and eat very little processed protein. These are essential nutrients for a healthy diet, and meat is a great source of high-quality protein to add to your diet. You should often include some protein in your meals or snacks.

Among the little industrially processed protein foods are: poultry, red meat, pork, eggs and dairy products. Choose products of organic origin if you want to avoid those that contain hormones or preservatives.

The proteins of vegetable origin that have undergone minimal treatment are: dried beans, lentils, even canned peas (as long as without added salt or in any case by rinsing and throwing the preservation liquid), frozen legumes without the addition of sauces or condiments. Tofu, tempeh, and seitan are plant-based proteins, but are generally considered more processed.

Among the partially industrially processed protein sources are: frozen meat without the addition of additives and sauces, natural yogurt and cheeses.

The foods that have undergone a significant transformation and that you must avoid are: cured meats, hot dogs, sausages, bacon, pre-cooked and then frozen meat or ready-made meat-based meals.

Buy and eat lightly processed grains

Whole grains are the best choice, which are very high in fiber and nutrients. However, not all whole grains are free from industrial treatments, so be careful.

The less processed ones you should focus on the most are: raw brown rice, quinoa, millet, whole wheat couscous and barley. Wholemeal pasta has undergone a major processing process, but it is a healthy supplement to your diet.

Do not buy precooked products, ready to heat in the microwave or that claim that can be cooked when in a hurry, because they have undergone further industrial processing to reduce preparation times at home.

You should also avoid refined grains such as rice, pasta and white bread, sweets, cakes and biscuits.

Once you have the right stock in the kitchen, you can start cooking your dishes without overly elaborate foods. Make sure that protein (poultry, red meat, pork, fish, low-fat dairy or legumes), fruits and vegetables form the basis of your meals.

An easy way to start cooking is to prepare the main course based on proteins. Add to this one or two ingredients, such as fruit, vegetables, or whole grains, to complete the meal.

Do not eat pre-made products such as prepackaged ones, frozen pizzas, pre-cooked meals, canned soups or pre-made sandwiches.

Have healthy snacks if allowed by your intermittent fasting protocol.

If you're hungry between meals, it's time for a snack. If you don't have a natural snack on hand, you'll be tempted to buy packaged ones, which are quick and easy. You should originally prepare healthy snacks to take with you at all times, to avoid overeating the industrially processed ones.

Try to have as many natural and healthy snacks with you as possible, if they are permitted by your intermittent fasting protocol. For example, have some fruit on hand (like apples), dried fruit or muesli prepared by yourself and take them to work. If you have the option to use a refrigerator, save certain foods, such as natural yogurt, raw vegetables, homemade hummus, or hard-boiled eggs.

Avoid typical processed snacks like candy, chips, crackers, snacks, packaged cake slices, single-serving cookies, or cereal / protein bars.

If you forget the snacks you made yourself at home or have no way to get them, at least look for the less processed snacks. For example, in many vending machines you will find packages of roasted peanuts or mixed nuts.

Don't go to fast food restaurants even on your cheat days

Many inexpensive or fast food restaurants offer a variety of highly processed foods. Although the menus have improved in recent years, it is still very difficult to find natural, whole and unprocessed foods.

Burgers, French fries, chicken nuggets, hot dogs, pizzas and other similar foods are just examples of food you usually find in cheap restaurants or fast food restaurants. Not only have these dishes undergone significant transformations, but if you eat them regularly they increase the risk of serious diseases, such as heart disease, hypertension and obesity.

If you still have to eat or choose fast food items, at least look for those products that are less processed and as natural as possible. For example, opt for a salad and grilled chicken, as they are the least processed ones you can order.

Eat processed foods in moderation. By eliminating or reducing processed foods from your diet you can control your weight and improve your overall health. However, an occasional snack or meal of processed products is allowed and should not cause serious adverse effects. Choose wisely and decide what "in moderation" really means to you.

If among your favorite foods there are some that have undergone an industrial process, you don't necessarily have to exclude them completely; for example, you can decide to eat them every Friday night or just once a month.

Remember that eliminating some industrial foods from your diet is still a great start. Ultimately, deciding how much or which processed food you want to exclude from your diet is essentially up to you.

Choose healthy alternatives

The most common processed foods are often also the tastiest. Think about what your favorites are (like sweets, pretzels, or crunchy biscuits) and consider if you can find a healthier alternative to replace them.

For example, if you want to eat something sweet after your meal, instead of choosing chocolate or ice cream, you can cut some fruit or eat plain yogurt with a little honey.

If you're craving something salty to munch on, grab a few carrots and bits of celery to eat with homemade hummus.

One of the most important tips we can give you is to prepare your favorite meals and snacks at home. In this way, you can keep track of what you eat without giving up good food.

Some easy ideas of snacks to have at home are: toppings, sauces or marinades, muesli or cereals, soups, stews and broths, baked foods such as muffins, cookies, granola bars, wholemeal bread or hummus.

If you wish, you can also prepare fast food-like meals at home. Homemade chicken nuggets and fries are definitely a better alternative than their restaurant versions.

Whatever you do, try to reduce the amount of processed food you have on a regulars basis and remember that a healthy intermittent fasting protocol prefers whole and natural foods.

Nancy Johnson

Conclusion

We would like to thank you for making it to the end of this book. We have done our best to ensure that every information contained is useful and helps you in your weight loss journey.

We know how frustrating it could be to start an intermittent fasting protocol and feeling discouraged by the fact that results do not appear immediately. As we repeated throughout the book, the goal of intermittent fasting is to create a healthy lifestyle that can support you over the years, not just give you a rapid decrease in weight.

By following the tips shared in this book, you will certainly burn fat, lose weight and feel much better. However, as we do not know you in person, our final recommendation can only be the following one.

Before starting an intermittent fasting protocol talk to your doctor and find out whether intermittent fasting could be a good idea for you or not. Remember, never sacrifice your health to fit into that new skirt you just got.

To your success!

Weight Loss for Beginners